अयुर्दा बलदा श्रीदा लोकप्रदानं न रिष्यति।
"May we have a long life, strength, and prosperity, and may it lead us towards greater good." - *Yajurveda*

With thanks and immense gratitude, first to the Creative Power of the Universe with whose Grace everything reaches fruition, next to the *Rishi Parampara*- the Seers responsible for maintaining continuity of eternal truths through the ages, and finally to the torch-bearers, mostly elderly women, who preserved and carried the knowledge of wellness forward and wove it into the fabric of Indian culture and life.

First edition 2024

We thank AI tools for support in generating all images.

Contents

Preface

The inspiration for this book comes from a glaring oddity. On the one hand we proudly claim to have longer life spans today and on the other, the number living with lifelong ailments is rapidly rising. The age at which ailments begin is also falling. More & more young are falling chronically sick.

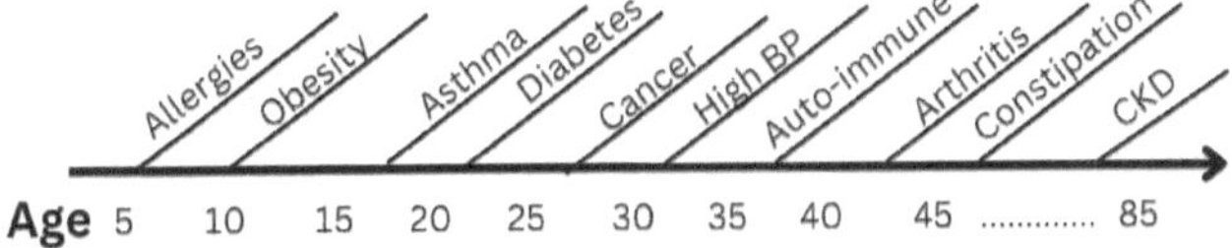

Is this acceptable? With the knowledge and means we have, one would think it is possible to live in good health for most part of our lives. Early and lifelong disease should be avoidable. The truth is, it is and this book is about learning how.

Ill-health like everything else, follows the law of action & consequence. It is a natural outcome of poor choices made knowingly or unknowingly. So the way to remove illness is simple: re-set the goals and priorities we chase.

Often the time spent in chasing takes us to a point where all the amassed wealth fails to restore health. We forget somewhere early on that a healthy person can easily acquire wealth and certainly enjoys better life. Lifestyle choices that support good health

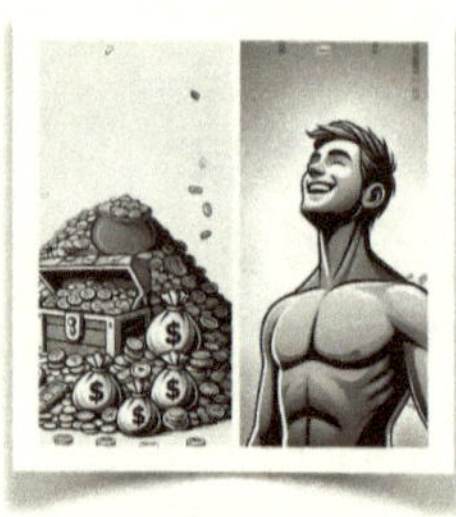

perhaps need to be prioritized sooner.

Are modern conveniences simplifying matter or are they misleading us? Do we understand the difference between living with managed conditions and being completely disease-free? By choosing what is convenient and not necessarily best for us, we agree to *get-by* in life with medicines. Should we instead be working to stay free and clear of illness and medicines, irrespective of age? Accepting a medicine-centered life compromises freedom. We cannot travel anywhere without the medicine box. In this context it is worth noting how animals move freely and stay healthy, given they also have physical bodies like humans.

Animals in natural habitats follow their instincts - *Ahar* (food to live), *Bhaya* (fear of protecting life), *Nidra* (proper sleep for rest & recuperation) and *Maithun* (sexual instinct for reproduction).

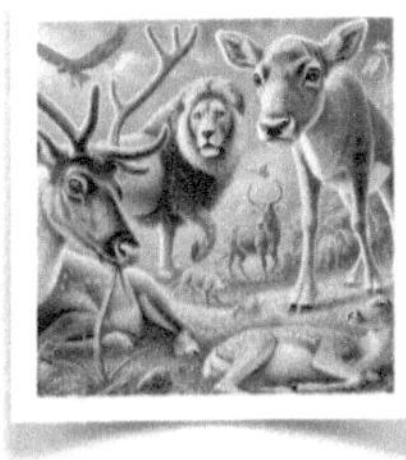

Following their cue, we can attain health and happiness abiding by standards prescribed by nature. We have the additional advantage of collective intelligence and learnings, all of which can be utilized to achieve superior levels of existence. Unfortunately, despite possessing the special power of intuition and intelligence, we misuse all the four instincts. Let us see how.

Today we choose to live to eat and not eat to live (*Ahar*), indulging in gluttony and putting fake foods in our body that is threatening our life. Not frightened about this, we instead live in constant fear (*Bhaya*) and non-stop worry about other unnecessary things. This deprives us of restful sleep (*Nidra*). In fact we spend many sleepless nights, uneasy, stressed and nervous. Reproductive organs are misused for enjoyment (*Maithun*) and over-indulgence. The result is loss of vigour & vitality, leading to sickness of the body.

Animals that live in natural habitats rarely fall sick. They do not have hospitals or doctors and are not dependent on medicines. They live freely and healthy by being close to nature and simply following their instincts. How do we miss this simple logic?

Unlike flora and fauna, human beings are out of sync with rhythms and cycles of nature, believing we are disconnected from our environment or that we can control nature. We consequently move into the slippery slope of ailments. We can move out of this 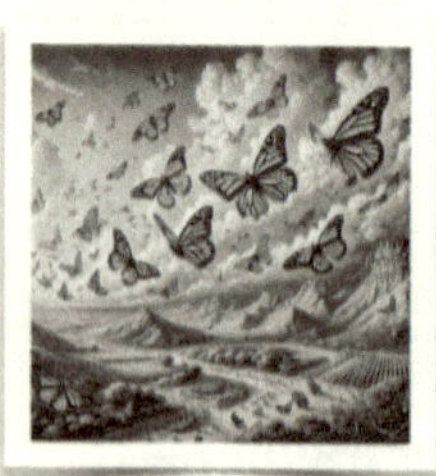 uncomfortable terrain and stay healthy till our last breath, provided we elect to understand and realign ourselves to these cycles. They are built into our body and are all around us.

Awareness of basic functions and anatomy also helps. Once we are empowered with this knowledge it is only a matter of time plus the effort we put to turn them into habits.

> **FOR GOOD HEALTH**
>
> *Align with Cycles of Nature*
>
> *Interconnect & Link with All Life*
>
> *Understand Basic Structure & Function of Body*
>
> *Be Aware of Supportive Techniques*

This book guides us to scientific techniques to stay healthy, lifelong. We simply support the body using these methods and it heals itself. Understanding is built with every chapter which have been kept short and succinct. Visuals along the way keep the journey easy and interesting.

The book starts with getting to know the silent, sentient machines in our body that work non-stop. The complete description of techniques is beyond the scope of this book but it provides enough so we can be well on our way towards disease reversal, if that indeed is what we want.

The first part of the book outlines physical ailments that many of us suffer from. It gets into their roots and throws light on the path to reversal. In part II we highlight practices to allay troubles of the mind i.e. how to maintain peak mental health. Understanding both physical and mental aspects, we will in times of trouble, know where to turn to for complete reversal of the problem.

It must be emphasized here that the book is not a diagnostic or treatment guide. Consulting a health practitioner is best suited for that. We just intent to present broad contours of wellness and point towards minor problems that are amenable to the self-help methods outlined in the book. The methods presented are taken from well-established holistic practices that the reader is advised to follow after due diligence. With that, we are positive that the book will provide the motivation to not just aim for, but *lead* a life that is vibrant and lived to its full potential.

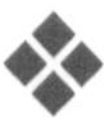

Part 1

1

Sentient Machines

The first step to good health is understanding the make up of our body, the sentient machines that work round-the-clock.

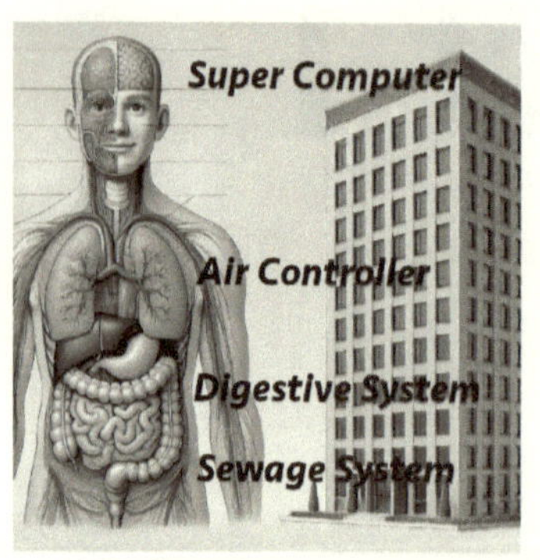

According to scientists, humans appeared on Earth more than 5 million years ago. The greatest wonder of creation made of ingenious living machines, the human body works skillfully to attain whatever it wishes. This delicate but strong frame can function in unbelievable harmony and work non-stop for more than a century. When trouble strikes, it can heal itself provided we support and not interfere with its processes. Let us look at this remarkable machine.

The human body is better than most modern, air-conditioned factories. It's 'building' has a sound structure built on strong pillars - legs and the spine which also give it movement. The *first floor*, which is up to the diaphragm, accommodates nutrition manufacturing (Digestive system), filtration as well as the sewage plant (Kidneys) to throw out waste. It also houses a unique reproduction plant. On the *second floor* of this human building there is a non-stop pump (Heart) and air-controllers (Lungs). The *top floor* is dome-shaped (Our Head) and accommodates the atomic reactor, a super-computer and telephone exchange (Brain) equipped with miles-long, exceedingly fast, communication system.

Amazingly, like a well designed transportation network where all locations are connected to each other, all the different plants work automatically in excellent co-ordination with one another. It is clear then that no system works in isolation, correct? Hence it is sub-optimal, even unscientific to design cures, assuming it is. Next, let us see why and how this interconnectivity exists.

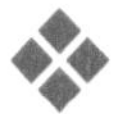

2

Building Blocks

The inter-dependent sentient motors in the body are an incredible feat of nature's engineering. We will now take a microscopic view and see up-close the building blocks of these magnificent organic machines built by nature.

From the modern science perspective, the cell is seen as the basic element. Holistic health sciences however, go deeper and explain how cells originate. They describe the forces that give birth to them.

There are five *subtle* forces that manifest as ether, air, fire, water and earth- the five *gross* elements (*Pancha Maha Bhutas*) that make up every cell in the body. In fact they are building blocks of all matter in this world. Each force is perceived by a sense organ.

The Five Forces

Subtle Forces [Tanmatras]	Gross Element [Mahabhuta]	Perceived by [Sense]
Sabda {Sound}	Ether / Akash	Ear
Sparsa {Touch}	Air / Vayu	Skin
Rupa {Form, Color}	Fire / Agni	Eye
Rasa {Taste}	Water / Apas	Tongue
Gandha {Smell}	Earth / Prithvi	Nose

Since all matter is made of the same five elements, it is easy to see the exchange of energy and connection between everything. All elements flow into each other. The water we drink comes from the rivers and goes back into it.

This might seem like a fantastic hypothesis. However, if we look around with a slight shift in perspective, we will see that this model explains clearly, why for example, imbalance in our water bodies (pollution, shortage) or cutting forests, impacts our health. It is because we are all connected! ***When our actions disturb the purity and balance of the five elements, can we expect to stay healthy?*** Some links may not be as noticeable especially if we live in cities, but that

does not make these strong ties mere imagination.
They are scientific truths that need to be sometimes perceived intuitively.

The Kaleidoscope of Life
The variety we see in this world is only multifarious ways in which the five elements combine and permutate to give rise to unique identities of matter. In other words, all forms of life have some combination of these elements.

Let us take the human body in which the five elements of nature are present in the following proportion:
Water - 72%
Earth - 12%
Fire   - 4%
Air   - 6%
Space - 6%

The elements express themselves as follows in various parts of the body.

Earth forms the solid structures such as teeth, nails, bones, muscles, skin, tissues, and hair. These give shape and strength to the body.
Water forms saliva, urine, semen, blood, and sweat.

Fire is represented in the digestive acids and enzymes that help convert food into energy. It forms the basis for hunger, thirst, sleep, vision in the eyes and complexion of the skin.

Air is responsible for all movement (physical and mental), expansion, contraction, vibration, and suppression.

Space is the most subtle of all elements and is present in the hollow cavities of the body. It represents the essential space needed by every organ and cell to function at its peak levels. It holds everything within itself and allows transmission of important signals, radio frequencies, light radiation and cosmic rays.

All holistic practices acknowledge the role of the five elements in maintaining health in the body. In Ayurveda, one of the most ancient and advanced life-sciences, instead of talking in terms of each of the five elements, all functions and processes taking place in the body are explained with reference to three biological forces called 'dosha.' *Vata* dosha is the force constituted by combination of ether and air; *Kapha* of earth and water and *Pitta* of fire and water.

If these five elements or three *dosas* are maintained in correct proportion in the body, proper metabolism is ensured and the body

remains healthy. Do we not trace every problem
in a machine or building to its constituent
materials? Just so, every disease in our body rises
from some impairment in its building blocks.

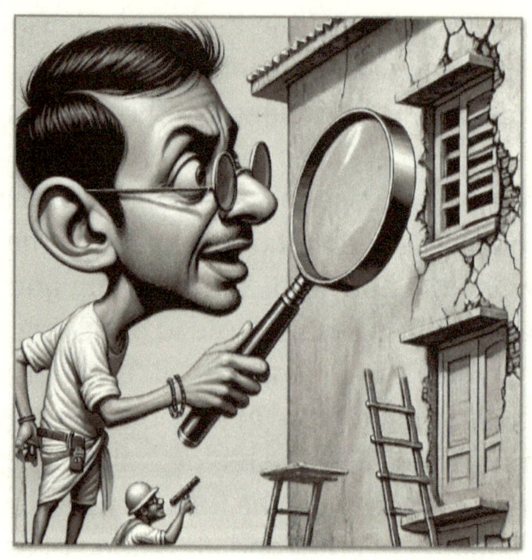

3

Root of Trouble

We can fix a problem in a machine only if we know which part is impacted and what caused the injury. Even though the immediate action is to fix the impacted part in the best way possible, in order to prevent the problem from recurring or growing in another part, we do need to get to the root of the trouble.

Since the building blocks of the body are the five elements, the root cause of every health problem is imbalance in the proportion of the five elements. In this chapter we will look at *how* imbalance in each element expresses itself as a disorder. The chapters that follow highlight some *ways to correct* the imbalance as well as present *causes* for the the imbalance. Understanding this we will be inspired to do regular cleansing as well avoid factors that lead to problems, both very important in the goal of maintaining good health.

Imbalance in the elements is expressed as deprecation (less) or aggravation (more) and either case expresses itself as disease. More than one element can be imbalanced at the same time and it is common to see existence of overlapping conditions attributable to imbalance in more than one element or *dosha*. Since we now recognize the role of each element and how they relate to the make up of our body, here are some examples where we can intuitively understand how excess or deficiency of an element causes certain diseases.

1. Imbalance of Earth Element

Excess Earth leads to issues like obesity, lethargy, congestion, high cholesterol, and 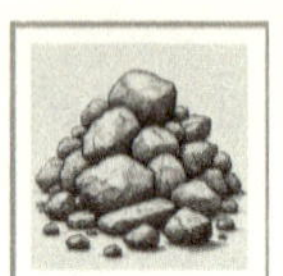 sluggish metabolism. Some diseases that result due to aggravated '*earth*' include sinus congestion, respiratory problems, and weight gain.

Deficient Earth can cause instability, lack of grounding, loose stools, weakness, poor digestion, anxiety, and weak immune function.

2. Imbalance of Water element

Excess Water causes fluid retention, edema, urinary problems, and excessive mucus. Diseases include 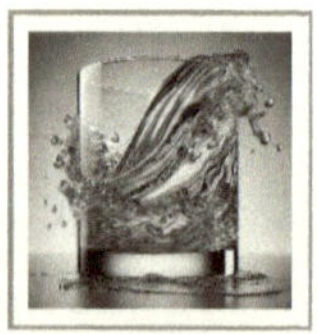

swollen joints, asthma, and heavy, damp
sensations in the body.
Deficient Water results in dehydration, dry skin,
constipation, back pain, and dry mucous
membranes.

3. **Imbalance of Fire element**

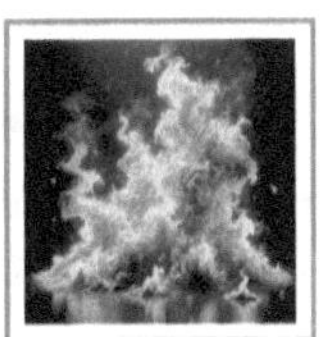

Excess Fire results in
inflammation, ulcers, acid reflux,
fever, anger, and irritability.
Diseases include gastritis, skin
disease, and hypertension.

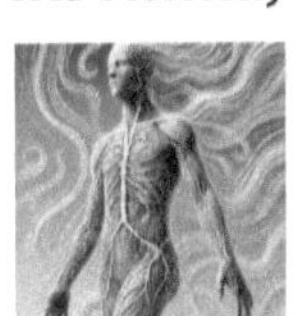

Deficient Fire leads to poor digestion,
slow metabolism, malnourishment
due to poor absorption of nutrients,
toxins in the body, lack of motivation,
and cold extremities.

4. **Imbalance of Air element**

Excess Air causes nervousness, dry skin,
insomnia, constipation, and joint pain. Diseases

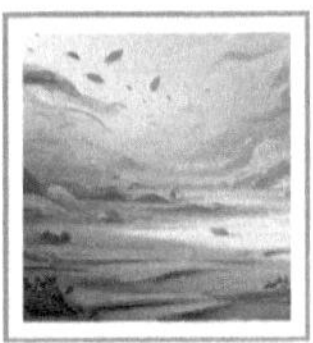

include arthritis, nervous system
disorders, and digestive issues.
Deficient Air results in
poor circulation, lack of
movement, blood
pressure problems, lung disorders,
depression, and stagnation in both
body and mind.

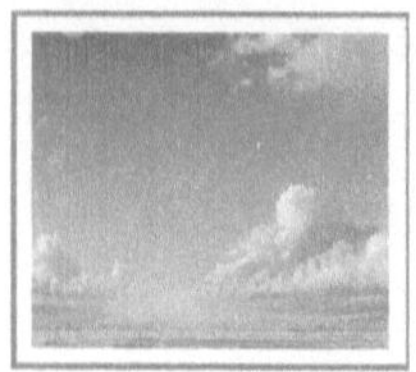

5. Imbalance of Space element
Excess Space can lead to speech disorders, epilepsy, madness, feeling ungrounded, anxiety, restlessness, and bloating.

Diseases include insomnia, anxiety disorders, and feeling disconnected.
Deficient Space might cause ear diseases, rigidity in thinking and feeling stuck, both physically and mentally.

As is evident, each element corresponds to specific body functions and emotional states. Physical and mental health issues are mere manifestations of imbalances in the elements. Balancing them is the right way to restore health.

Q: How do we balance them?
A: Manipulate the elements themselves. Which means change diet and lifestyle.
Q: How is that so?
A: Food which is part of our environment embodies the same five elements. In order to remedy the imbalance all we need to do is choose foods that add the missing elements and reduce those in excess in our body.

Likewise, incorrect lifestyle, disturbed sleep cycle, and sedentary habits disturb the elements and upset metabolism. Being sluggish slows down circulation and movement of air and water (blood) which is key to nutrient and oxygen flow. As importantly, it slows down elimination of morbid and toxic waste which can in itself become a cause of disease. Reversing disease is a matter of adopting right diet and lifestyle and recovery is hastened by stopping entry to toxic materials and utilizing appropriate therapeutic techniques.

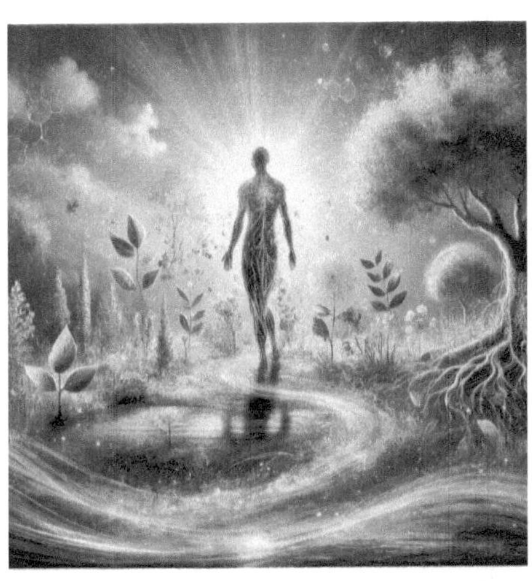

The body is designed by nature to move towards balance. The symptoms we see - fever, cough, vomit, cold, loose motions- are all signs of the body trying to expel what it sees as an intruder or a trouble-maker disturbing with the balance. Suppressing symptoms with drugs goes against natural design. This does not mean we do nothing. There are many therapeutic systems that alleviate symptoms *along with* restoring lost elemental balance, which go in step with nature's healing design.

What are the techniques that support this natural healing design?

Practices that embody the knowledge of the elements and its universality. Naturopathy, Ayurveda and other holistic health sciences have fully developed understanding of the connections between elements and all life. They restore proper flow of energy in the body, freeing us from expensive and undesirable effects of drug dependency. Modern medicine specialize in stopping body's processes with aggressive use of NSAIDs, antibiotics, steroids and surgery, usually in that order. Holistic practices nurture positive forces that support effective healing. An expert in them may also be equipped to dispense urgent care. We will now touch some of these powerful therapeutic techniques in the following chapters and marvel at their science.

4

Nature Cures

Nature by design cures and moves towards balance. Since our body is designed by Nature, it too moves towards balance. Naturopathy is the science that enumerates the tools of Nature that anyone can use in supporting cure of disease. Since the body is made of the five elements, naturopathy deploys them (viz. earth, water, fire, air and space) skillfully to eliminate toxins from the body. With cleansing done, the power and flow of life current is restored which enables the body to heal itself. Disease is thereby cured. Efficient function and balance is reestablished in a natural way without causing further disruption in the body.

Here are some examples of how the elements are used to cleanse and purify the body along with a few instances of conditions they are helpful in. Some of these can be easily performed at home and used also as periodic cleansing practices in the interest of preventing maladies. However, if a serious condition exists, it is best to use them under able guidance.

EARTH

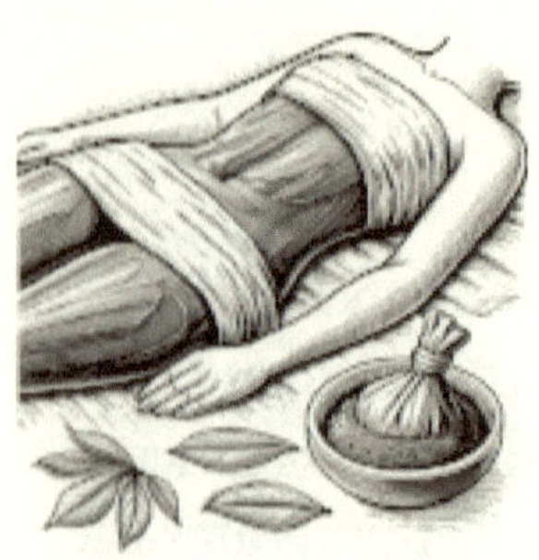

Cleansing through earth is done by placing **wet mud packs** on the affected parts. If proper mud is not available, the **paste of green plants** like basil, moringa or mint can be applied. Such a pack can be put on the stomach and skin. For better results, after applying green pack, the body can be directly exposed to sun rays or blue light. The results are wonderful for constipation and skin diseases like white spots.

WATER

Water is used for hydration, making hot and cold packs and for flushing out waste through enema.

Drinking adequate amounts of water - 8 to 10 glasses every day ensures cells are washed and hydrated. The water should ideally be kept in a copper vessel overnight or for 8-10 hours. Since it is difficult to clean the copper vessel daily, a glass or steel vessel can be used with a clean (about 3"x 8") copper plate

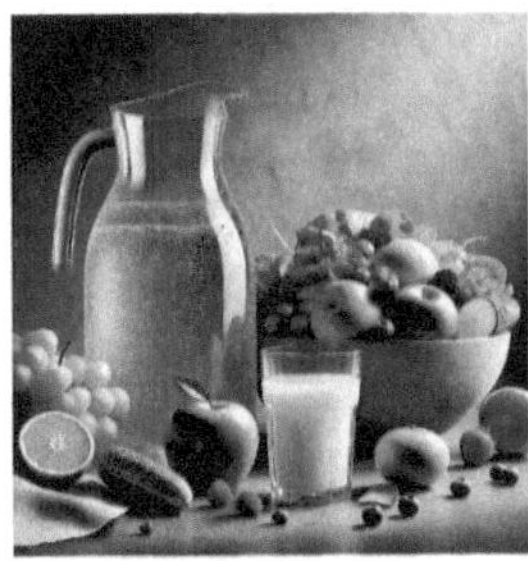

dipped in it. This water, called **structured water**, is best used for drinking as well as cooking. It draws out toxins from cells, pulling them naturally towards itself and expelling via urine. After drinking 2 or 3 glasses in the morning, walk for 10 minutes before going to the toilet. This practice helps to get rid of constipation and excess heat which is the reason for many diseases. <u>Sufficient hydration can be ensured through the day with a combination of water, fresh juices, fruit and raw vegetables/ salads</u>.

Note: Make sure the copper plate is cleaned with tamarind paste daily. Scrubbing with mix of lemon juice and salt to add shine is optional.

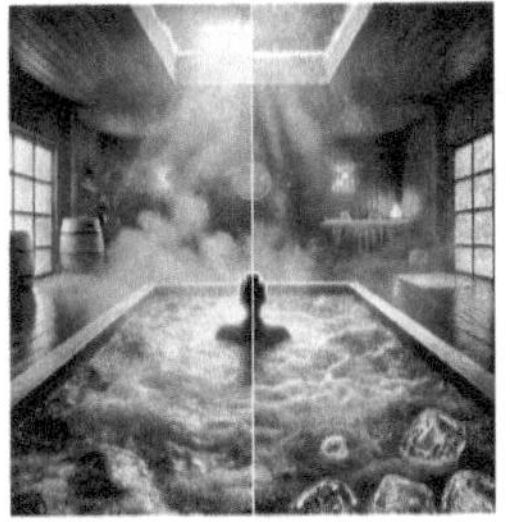

Hot and cold packs with water help in reducing fever and removing toxins from the body.

Hot therapy increases blood flow to the area, relieves pain and swelling in case of sore muscles, joints or fever.

How to make and when to use a hot pack?

1. Dip a cotton bed sheet or towel in hot water.

2. Wring out excess water

3. Wrap around the body. Cover with woolen blanket or plastic for 15 to 30 minutes.

For smaller areas, a hot water bottle can also be used instead of towel. This can be repeated after 1 or 2 hours, if necessary.

Cold Pack is helpful for injuries, inflamed joints and for placing on stomach to remove waste. It constricts blood vessels and numbs to reduce pain.

The same process is followed as in hot therapy, except use ice or cold water to dip the towel. Wring and apply on the area. Leave on for 15-20 minutes.

Combination of hot and cold therapy can be used, repeating the hot-cold cycle for 3-5 minutes each, to enhance circulation and reduce pain

Enema

Water dissolves and washes away waste. This fact is used to remove garbage from the large intestine. With or without constipation, this

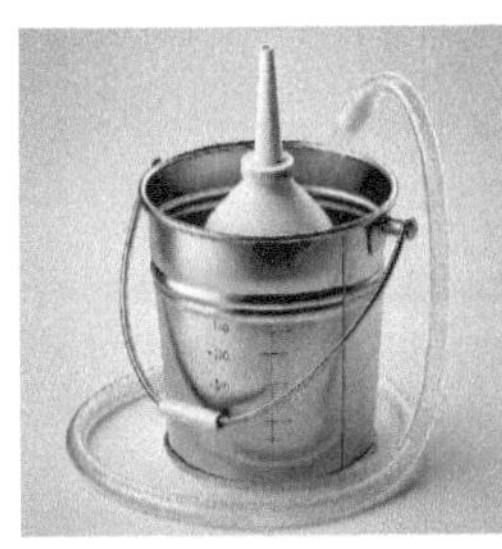

simple technique, done periodically and especially during fasting has an intensely purifying effect on the whole body. That is because <u>the gut is the fuel center and second brain</u>. It is thus imperative to keep it clean. Enema is helpful in preventing colon cancer by stopping waste from sticking to the gut, hardening and distorting the perfectly shaped elimination pipes. <u>Holistic health sciences have always recognized the gut-brain connection</u> and with current research corroborating this link, it is now easier to appreciate why holistic health sciences focus on gut cleansing as the first step to healing any condition. Setting the gut right and cleaning it leads to improved brain signaling and therefore functioning of the entire body.

Enema should be done with lukewarm water. One spoon of castor oil can be added to the water for better results. Ayurveda also offers medicinal herbs that can be used under guidance. Once learnt, an enema kit can be kept at home and this technique can be easily done in the comfort of one's home with excellent results.

FIRE

Fire in the body refers to energy in the cell and gastric fire needed for proper digestion, assimilation and energy. It is essential to have sufficient amounts of digestive juices in the body at every age. The stomach acid and digestive enzymes continue secreting optimally if the organs are stimulated via proper body movement, acupressure or massage. In view of the sedentary lifestyle of many, it is absolutely necessary to include some physical exercise daily for an hour. It can be walking, jogging, yoga, or a mix of movements. Specific foods also contribute to fueling this fire. These must be part of our diet and we will learn about them in the following sections.

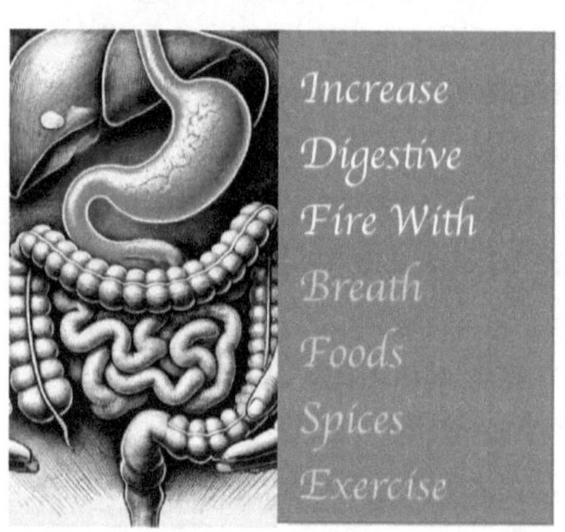

There is also a 'bad' kind of fire or excess heat that must be removed from the body. It is directly related to inflammation. There are other natural ways but drinking sufficient water and taking bath twice every day (especially in Indian summer) is the simplest way to remove excess heat from the body. The bad heat of inflammation has to be calmed by zeroing into the culprit causing it (for example, preservative & additives) and removing it from the body and stopping its entry subsequently. Kitchen spices as we will see later also help in removing this excess heat.

AIR

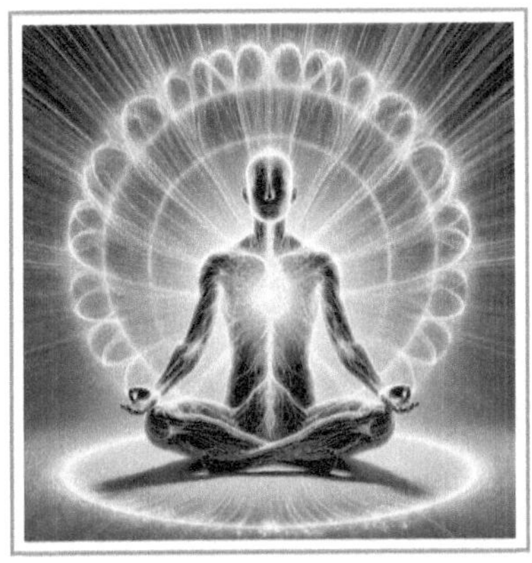

Pure air is a great doctor. Inhaling fresh air walking early morning and evening is well known. Methods of *Pranayama* can be learnt easily and done for minimum of 15 minutes daily. It is a scientific fact that *prana* or energy flow is foundational. The body exists as long as *prana* flows in it. Breathing exercises and techniques vitalize the body even more than the diet we take. Recharging the body with air, morning and evening is essential for good health.

SUN (SPACE)

In our quest for convenient pills for every ailment, we have ironically forgotten Nature's most expedient gift- the sun. All living beings get their energy from the sun. This energy is abundant, unlimited and should be harnessed to the maximum.

The sun looks white, but consists of seven colours viz. violet, indigo, blue, green, yellow, orange and red (VIBGYOR). Of these, the first three have a cooling effect on the body and are also antiseptic. Green is neutral. The last three colours create heat. Using colour as therapy is called Chromotherapy and is part of nature-cure science. In naturopathy, chromotherapy is used to cure chronic and dreaded diseases. Here are some examples:

White is full spectrum light and is purifying. It is used to bring balance and clarity and helpful in treating SAD (Seasonal Affective Disorder). Simply exposing ourselves to the sun at the right time (3 hours within sunrise and sunset) fortifies Vitamin D in the body and uplifts our mood.

Red is stimulating and improves circulation. It is used to increase blood flow and thereby energize the body.

Blue is calming and helpful in treating stress, sleeplessness and high blood pressure.
Other colors also have their beneficial effects. One can use color in clothing, wall-paint, light, flowers and visualization to benefit from their healing frequencies.

Therapeutic water can be easily made by using colored glass bottles or plain glass covered in appropriate colored cellophane sheets and sunning them for a day. This water can then be used after naturally cooling it in the evening.

Fasting

In the nature cure system, fasting is another powerful method for keeping the body healthy throughout. <u>Fasting or skipping one meal, once a week, removes toxins in the digestive organs</u>. This fact received the Nobel prize in 2016 but has been recognized for centuries in holistic sciences including Ayurveda. If new to fasting, it can be started by drinking only water, green juices or mono fruit juices.

Naturopathy Treatment

There are nature cure hospitals in almost every country. Use the powerful internet search engines to locate one in your area. One can take treatment in these hospitals or join them to learn nature cure methods and follow them at home to prevent sickness.

Prevention is the best approach to staying healthy. It is interesting in this context that some nature-cure hospitals now offer a week-long 'human body servicing package' for cleaning the body annually. If we find it hard to do it ourselves it is a perhaps a good idea to get periodic purification done. Just as it is with *Panchakarma* in Ayurveda, cleaning equals preventing disease. We <u>need</u> to keep our house clean to allow proper function, similarly our body needs to stay clean to perform at its best.

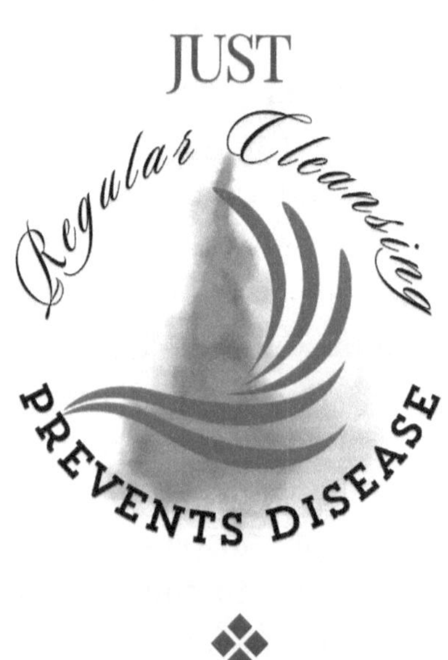

5

Defining 'Health'

To get health right, we have to first define it correctly. Where else but in the oldest science of life, Ayurveda, can we find its precise understanding?

Unlike most other practices, the concept of health or *swastha* in Ayurveda goes beyond the simple *absence* of disease. It defines health as:

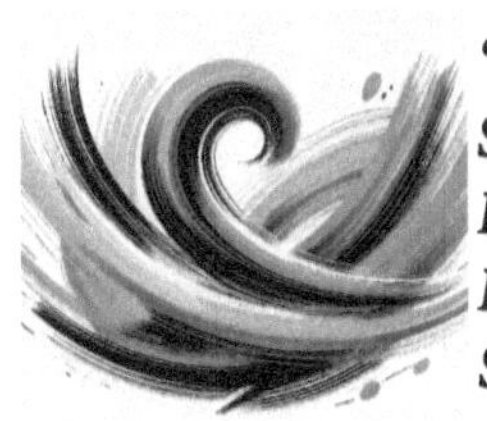

"SAMA DOSHA SAMA AGNISHCHA SAMADHATU MALA KRIYAAHA| PRASANNA ATMA MANA INDRIYAHA SWASTHA ITI ABHIDHEEYATE ||

This *sloka* or Sanskrit verse is quoted from *Sushruta Samhita,* written in 600 B.C by Sushruta, the world's first surgeon. Let us understand the elements in the definition.

Sama Dosha means balanced or in equilibrium *Dosha.*

Doshas as mentioned in chapter 2 are the energetic forces - *vata, pitta and kapha. Vata,* a combination of air and space elements, *Pitta* of fire and water and *Kapha* of earth and water. Every body has some *dosha* dominant in them and even though the balance and composition of each *dosha* varies from person to person, all three must be in a balanced state in every person, at all times, to maintain a state of good health. As we know already, when the balance is disturbed- either aggravated or decreased (vitiated)- it sets the stage for development of disease.

Sama Agni means balanced 'Fire.'

In Ayurveda the imbalance in digestive fire (*Agni*) is one of the primary causes for most diseases. Ayurveda defines *Agni* not only as digestive fire, but the energy behind *all* metabolic processes of the body. Hence balanced fire is critical to maintaining good health.

Sama Dhatu means balanced tissues.

Ayurveda defines seven *dhatus* or tissues in our
body.
Rasa - nutritive fluid
Rakta - blood
Mamsa - muscle
Meda - fat
Asthi - bones
Majja - bone marrow
Shukra - ovum & sperm
Wellness is synonymous with balanced state of all
dhatus (tissues).

Mala Kriya is waste elimination process.
The waste system or *Malas* includes elimination
of *Purisa* (stools), *Mutra* (urine) and, *Sweda*
(sweat). All must function daily for good health.

Prasanna Atma Mana Indriya:
Prasanna is experiencing satisfaction or
contentment.
Atma or *jiv atma* is the individual soul.
Indriya is sense organs through which we
experience the world we live in.
Mana is the mind and is seen as an incredible tool
that must be trained and sharpened.

Putting it together: the soul, senses and mind
must be in a state of satisfaction, joy and peace.

Summarizing the three lines, a healthy person is someone whose *doshas, agni, dhatus and mala kriya* are in a balanced state, and the mind (*mana*), sense organs (*indriyas*), and -soul (*atma*) is in a pleasant state (*prasanna*).

SWASTHA ITI ABHIDHEEYATE

Now the last line of the definition. *Swastha* means good health. The word however, can be broken down into two roots that make it. 'S*wa*' means 'self' and '*stha*' means 'situated, located or anchored'. Taken together it means we are in good health when we are concurrently anchored to or established in our self. This is a seemingly philosophical perspective because it takes into account non-physical dimensions of the body.

Iti Abhidheeyate means 'thus so, upon contemplation'. Sushruta thus spells clearly that after deep study one can state that good health is ascertained only when there is a global state of balance in the body. Along with that the mind, senses and soul must experience joy and be situated in the self. Only when all the above is true a person experiences well being and bliss.

The science of Ayurveda proposes a vision of the individual that encompasses the often overlooked holistic aspects of the mind & soul that modern science is slowly beginning to acknowledge.

Ayurveda is a huge body of science and a treasure trove of knowledge. There are many suggestions and procedures within the corpus of Ayurveda that one can apply easily at home without gaining complete expertise and a seeker who embarks to learn it is well rewarded.

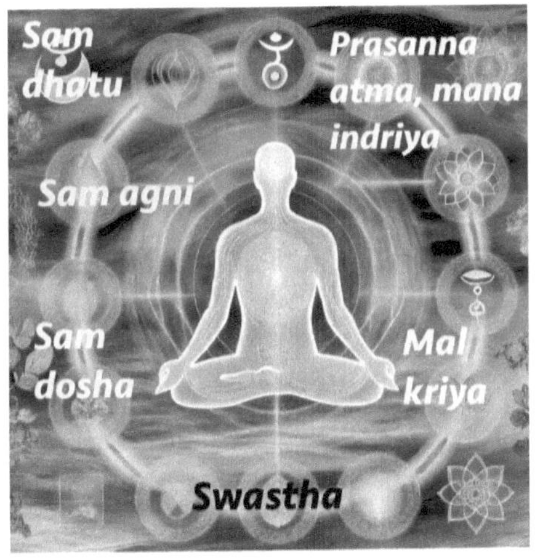

Iti

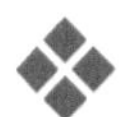

6

Switches on Our Body

Nature has placed many switches on our body that when pressed, signal the part connected to it to wake up and work properly. These switches are captured in the science of Acupressure.

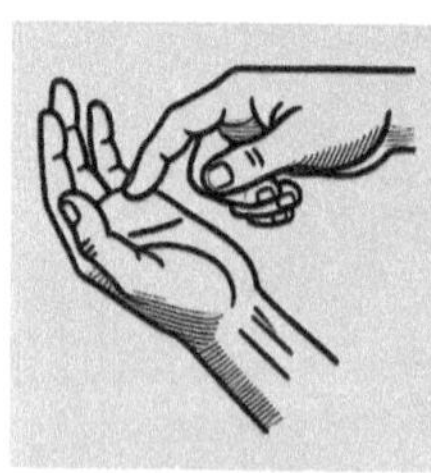

Acupressure therapy is yet another offspring of Nature's science and an invaluable gift to humankind. Just as Nature's bounty - sunshine, air and water- is bestowed generously, this therapy can be harnessed by anyone for maintaining, even restoring good health.

The word acupressure is related to acupuncture. *Acu* is derived from Latin and Greek origins and means 'needle' or 'point' and *puncture* means to pierce. Just as acupuncture is the art of treating disease by piercing a needle in specific points on the body, similarly acupressure is the art of healing by applying pressure on specific points

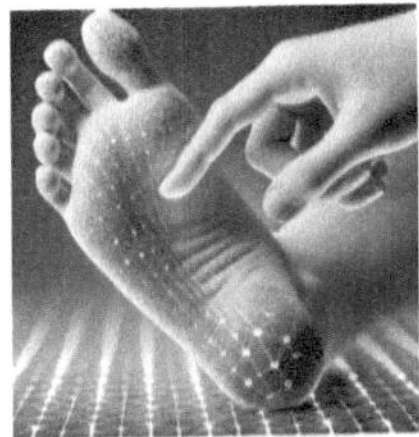

with the help of one's thumb or unpointed things.

This science represents built-in wisdom in the human body and offers easy therapeutics via impulses sent to desired parts of the body. The start-up switches (points) for each organ of the body are available in the palms and soles. One has only to identify these switches under the guidance of an experienced teacher.

The strength of this technique lies in its simplicity. It merely involves giving pressure on the point which represents an organ and repeat it three times a day. The treatment is continued till the pain on these points subsides.

There is three-pronged benefit to acupressure.

1. **Prevention of all types of diseases**: By pressing the points for about 10 minutes, the relative organs are activated and recharged like a battery cell and all the endocrine glands are normalized. The end result is proper alignment

and function of organs and glands that
preempts and corrects disease.

2. **Instant diagnosis without any laboratory
tests**: If there is pain on or around a point on
pressing, it indicates a problem with the organ
connected with that point. Since disease in any
organ or part of the body is reflected in the
corresponding point of the palms or soles, this
therapy is also called 'Reflexology'. When there
is pain, it is said in the language of electricity
that the 'fuse' is off in that part. Thus one can
diagnose disease instantly without costly
laboratory tests.

3.**Cure for diseases**: The cure is
straightforward. Apply pressure intermittently
like a pump for two minutes on the point where
it hurts. Repeat this treatment three times
during 24 hours. The motto of Acupressure is :
If you feel pain, press it out.

Acupressure point charts are easily available in
many places and can be slowly memorized.
Acupressure on the self can be then turned into
an easy to do, daily habit.

Related to Acupressure is another non-invasive,
medicine-free treatment known as

Neurotherapy. It is also called *Nadi Mardan Kriya* or nerve manipulation procedure. It is based on Vedic knowledge of *nadis* or energy channels combined with understanding of anatomy and physiology. Designed by Lajpat Rai Mehra, this system of healing relies on stimulating organs and tissues in a specific way, using the right amount of pressure on different parts of the body. This triggers proper function, release and absorption of essential enzymes, vitamins and catalysts that restores balance. Neurotherapy has successfully healed many serious conditions dismissed as un-treatable by modern medicine. While there are some self-help techniques in the practice, it is better to seek guidance to experience the benefits of this remarkable modality.

With its ease, simplicity and almost total lack of tools, acupressure and neurotherapy are great therapies within reach of every person. With just a little practice and regularity they can be immensely useful to improve and maintain overall wellness. Both the systems are completely devoid of negative side-effects and combined with corrective diet, go the right way in reversing ill health.

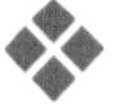

7

Yoga-Link to the Universe

First and foremost, let us clear the confusion about various styles of yoga doing the rounds across the world - Ashtanga yoga, Hatha yoga, Hot yoga, Iyengar yoga, Kundalini yoga, Power yoga, Restorative yoga, Vinyasa yoga, etc.

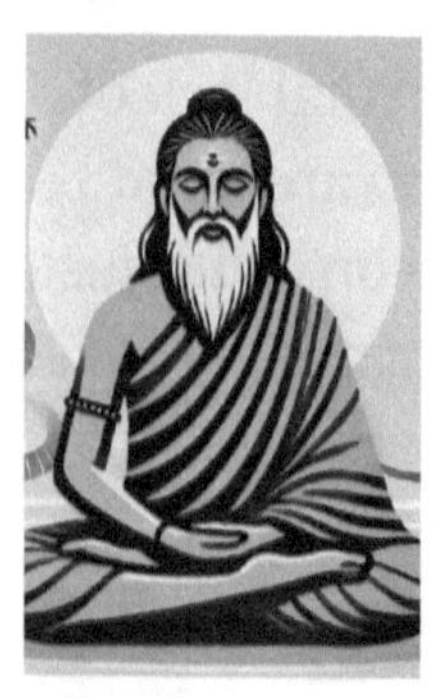

Understanding of Yoga comes from two cardinal sources. One is *Yoga Sutras* of **Sage Patanjali**. This is a collection of 195 Sanskrit *sutras* or verses on the theory and practice of yoga. The time the *sutras* were compiled in India by sage Patanjali is uncertain- any time after the turn of the Common Era (first to the second century) to several centuries before that.

He assembled and organized the knowledge of yoga from multiple older traditions. His text refers to the eight limbs of yoga viz. *Yama, Niyama, Asana, Pranayama, Pratyahara, Dharana, Dhyana and Samadhi*. Hence the practice of Yoga that spread from it is called *Ashtanga*

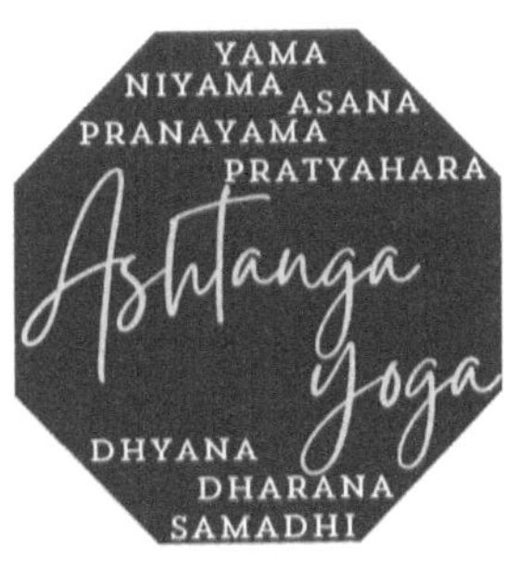

(eight limbs) Yoga.

The second source of yoga knowledge is *Hatha* Yoga by Swami Svatmarama whose book *HathaYoga Pradipika* is a fifteenth century classic Sanskrit manual.

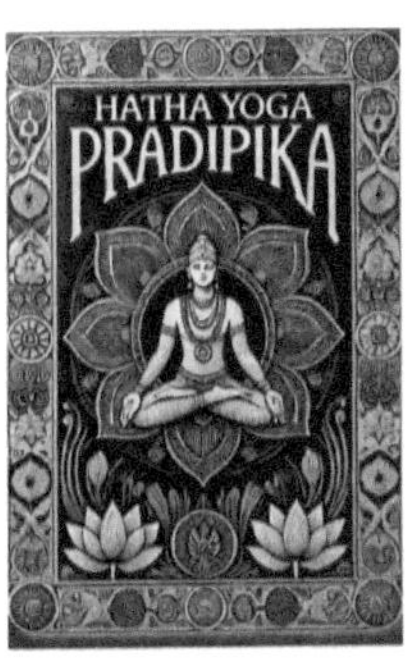

Ha-tha refers to sun and moon corresponding to right and left nostril breath with which purification, balance and bliss is attained through practice of *asana*, *bandha*, concentration, *mudra*, *pranayama* and *shatkarma*.

All other yoga styles are rooted in these two ancient texts and carry distinct appeal factors since they have been developed by different people responding to exigences of society, culture and marketing.

The word **Yoga** itself means 'union' - that of the mind with the soul and also of the soul with divinity. By clearly defining the goal as well as the path to it, *yoga* signifies both means and the end. Even as benefits are experienced along the way, once this union is attained, a state of perfection is achieved.

Power of Intuition

Some aspects of *Yoga* have been researched and their merits chronicled in scientific journals.

However, many facets of this ancient body of knowledge like soul, *prana-shakti*, *nadis* and *chakras* (energetic channels and vortexes) have to be grasped intuitively since they remain beyond reach of 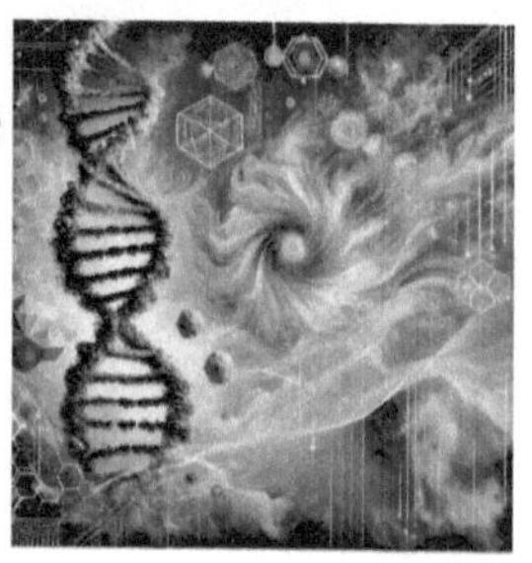 modern tools. Be that as it may, they are time-tested truths and available for all to experience. *Yoga* thus can be seen as situated in both art and science.

We must realize though, separating disciplines into art and science, like the brain into left and right side, is only a matter of convenience and organization. Life processes are a blend of art and science just as cognitive tasks engage both sides of the brain. We perceive many things intuitively. That modern science is as yet unable to explain everything is a reflection of our limitations. It does not mean we dismiss what we cannot explain or sense physically. Giving more weight to the sequential logic and rejecting intuition is limiting and detrimental. It has unfortunately led to many misunderstandings and exclusion of valuable therapies. In fact, it is unscientific to dismiss holistic practices that take into account fundamental connections and realities, and call them 'psuedo-science.' They work, with great economy and technique, even if inexplicable.

No Room for Disease

Yoga goes beyond bending and stretching of limbs in various postures. It is not just ringing a bell, staring at a candle or looking at a dot on the wall. These are only preliminary aids or techniques used in the whole corpus of yoga.

Yoga is embracing a lifestyle. All diseases–physical, mental, emotional– are reversed as a natural fallout. The journey gradually refines our personality, aligning it closer with the laws of the universe.

There is no room for disease with such alignment.

Decisions with Clarity

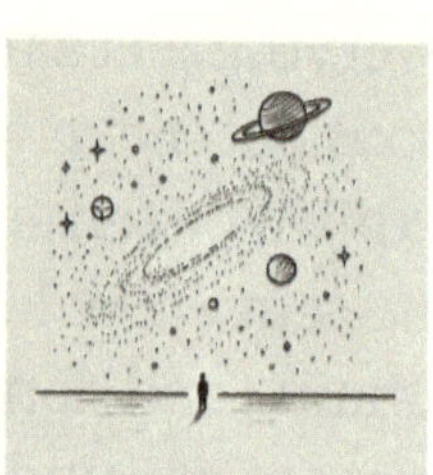

Practicing yoga, we realize our position in the order of things. Once we know our place, we know what to do in every situation with no special instructions needed when faced with a decision. The right choice to make in any given condition - simple to complex-becomes intuitively evident.

For example, hunger will give us the answer to eat or not; in responding to an angry person we will be lead to the source and real target of the anger; when faced with the decision to use an untested or harmful chemical, the rejection will be automatic because the thought of harm to other life forms will rise naturally. Clarity in mind - a consequence of yoga- will lead us to right choices and decisions under the circumstance.

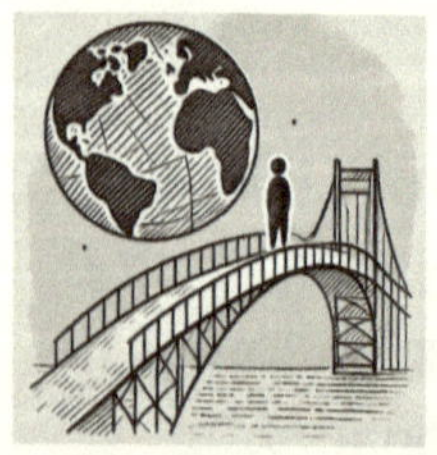

Building Bridges

Ignorance is our main affliction. Ignorance about our own body and its connection to the universe. Ignorance based on disjointed view of things confers erroneous pleasures because it fosters a misguided sense of satisfaction, leading us to believe all is well and nothing is amiss. Yoga draws the bridges to things that we otherwise fail to see as connected. For example, when we see the domino effect of our actions it changes the way we use our resources like rivers and lakes. We are more careful in our use and about polluting them .

What we lack today is not resources- money, buildings, or lands- so much as right knowledge. Intelligence that aids us to manage daily affairs and crisis in a patch-work manner differs from cultivating the wisdom essential for navigating life in its totality with all its simplicities and complexities.

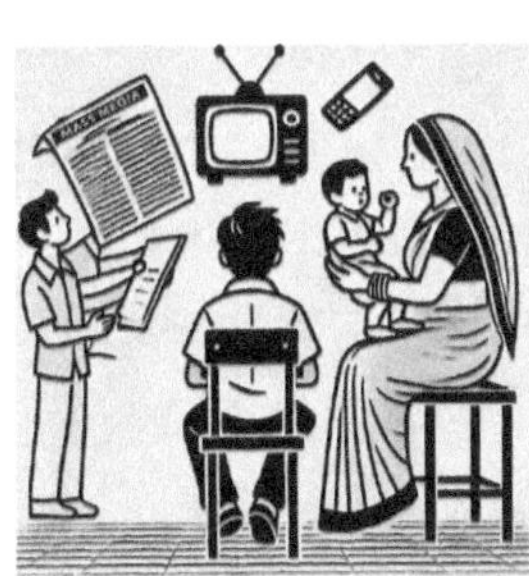

Make-Over of the Mind

A conditioned mind is unfit for yoga. Our ideas and perspectives get influenced by our social milieu and circumstances. We first learn about things from our parents, then school teachers followed by society, media, culture, geography, et al. We do not realize when stereotypes or pre-conceived notions set in and begin to color the way we see and understand things. Only when we see follies in our thinking and know that we do not know or know wrong, we are driven to change and recondition our mind.

In order to practice yoga we have to shed the conditioning started right from childhood.

Coding the Cell

Biology tells us that we started from a single cell.
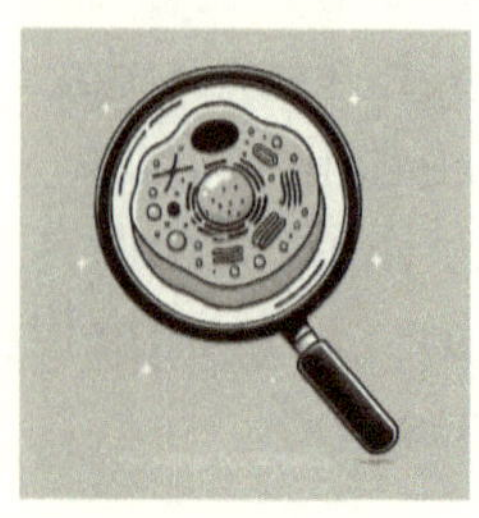
This one cell split into two to give a bi-cell, then into four to give a quarter cell, and so on. A mono cell is thus the origin of the large human body. Science tells us that if this little cell was analyzed minutely it could tell us how long the body evolving from it would live, the experiences it would pass through, and every other detail till the death of the individual. It is all programmed into this little cell. It thus becomes crucial that the intelligence in the cell is mapped correctly. Epigenetics touches this subject and the science of yoga shows the way to code the right intelligence so that we can live a healthy life.

In addition to reconditioning the mind and allowing us to see our position in the universe, with the *yama, niyama, and pratyahara* aspects, let us see *how* yoga practice helps us code intelligence correctly in the cells to keep us in good health.

A*sana* (physical postures), *pranayama* (breathing techniques), and d*hyana, dharana, samadhi* (contemplation, focus and deep meditation), lay the foundations for wellness by coding. We can consider *dhayna, dharna* and *samadhi* together as meditation for our purposes here. The great news is that a*sana, pranayama* and *meditation* is beneficial and accessible to all age-groups.

Asanas: The practice of yoga asanas develops strength, flexibility, recoding memory in muscles, while soothing the nerves and calming the mind. Asanas affect the whole body- muscles, bones, joints , skin, glands, nerves, and internal organs.
Pranayama: Controlled, deep and mindful breathing in pranayama relaxes the mind and reduces stress stimuli. On the physical level, pranayama clears airway secretions, enhances respiratory muscle function and increases lung capacity. Repeated practice of various techniques help us get a handle on our emotional response to stimuli and stop disease in its roots. The effects of pranayama go deep into the cells and greater realizations can be attained pursuing the study of *Swara* (dominant nostril) *Yoga.*

Meditation: Meditation increases self-awareness and sense of purpose. It increases benefits initiated by pranayama manifold providing insights on how to <u>respond</u>, rather than <u>react</u> to situations in life. Ultimately it helps to build cell resilience and improve mental and emotional well-being.

With regular practice started early in childhood the natural consequence of yoga is a strong immune system, improved flexibility and posture, healthy joints, optimal blood pressure, weight, stress, and composure. With the system in balance the cumulative effect is slow down in the aging process and increased ability to go through vicissitudes of life with peace and grace.

Learning Yoga: It is necessary to practice and learn yoga from an expert. To avail benefits from this time-tested science of the human body, sufficient and regular time must be put in, as per individual requirement. If motivation and discipline exist, yoga can be mastered fairly easily. Once embraced there is only progress, growth, joy and greatly improved quality of life.

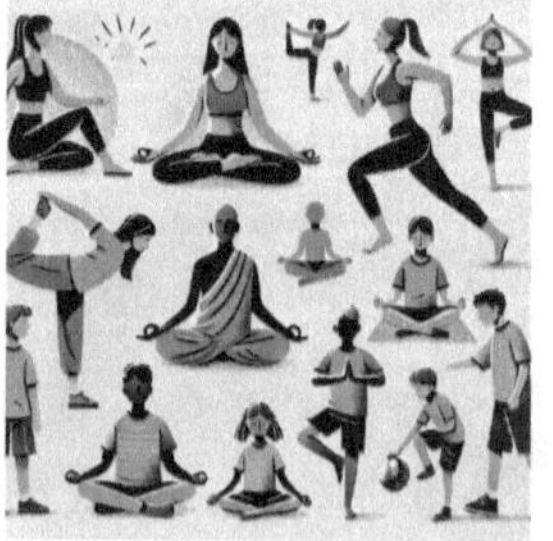

8

Flow & Glow

Oil massage is a therapeutic practice that involves the application of warm oils to the body using special massage techniques. It is part of Ayurveda and Naturopathy but included here

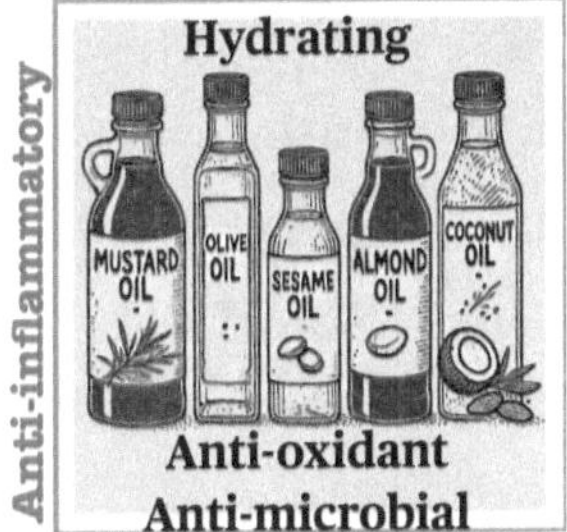

for its stand alone benefits and ease of use on a regular basis by anyone.

A good massage helps detox as well as calm both the body and the mind. It heals physically, mentally, alleviates muscular tension, reduces stress and improves overall health. This age old practice has been valued across various cultures for its numerous merits and is used globally for relaxation, healing, and rejuvenation. Call it flow and glow therapy if you please.

The choice of massage oil can significantly amplify the virtuous effects of massage. Traditionally, mustard, coconut and sesame oil is used in India for massage and often infused with medicinal herbs. All the three oils are excellent choices. While mustard is better in colder climes, sesame and coconut are preferred in warmer areas. Other oils used in different parts of the

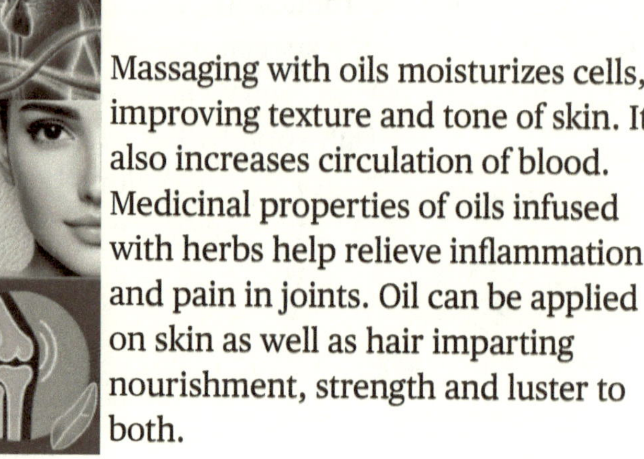

world include jojoba, almond, olive, marula, and argan.

Massaging with oils moisturizes cells, improving texture and tone of skin. It also increases circulation of blood. Medicinal properties of oils infused with herbs help relieve inflammation and pain in joints. Oil can be applied on skin as well as hair imparting nourishment, strength and luster to both.

Benefits

Bull driven or Ghani oils are the best oils to use. Cold pressed are the next choice if Ghana oils are not easily available. Most oils provide great benefits but since sesame oil is one of the most favored oil for massage here is a list of few of its merits.

1. Sesame oil is loaded with antioxidants which helps in *eliminating environmental stressors - toxins and harmful free radicals from the body. It is thus a powerful cleansing agent and excellent for purifying the skin.

2. The antimicrobial properties of sesame oil *prevent the growth of harmful germs*, thereby keeping the skin healthy and free of infection.

3. Sesame oil is rich in anti-inflammatory compounds helping in conditions like arthritis and wound healing.

4. Sesame oil shields the skin from the harmful ultraviolet rays of the Sun and acts as a natural sunscreen. Regular, simply topical use of sesame oil with aloe vera gel is helpful in protecting the skin while at the same time allowing exposure to Sun for Vitamin D.

5. Just as it is important to drink sufficient water to keep the body hydrated from within, it is equally essential to keep the skin moisturized from the outside. A massage with sesame oil penetrates the skin to hydrate its lower layers and prevents dryness, formation of scaly skin texture and rashes and itching caused due to dryness.

'Massaging' the teeth, gums and oral cavity with sesame oil by oil-pulling for 15-20 minutes daily ensures strength and health of both the teeth and gums. Adding clove, turmeric and salt to the oil prevents gum disease as well as heals gingivitis.

Cost of Treating Gum Disease	
Regular Dentist	*Sesame Oil-Pulling*
US $ 1000+	<US $ 10

Massaging with oils tailored to individual needs is a marvelous way to connect with one's body and mind. Good quality oils, extracted the right way, generally provide a wide spectrum of benefits. They can be self-applied to gain protection from pathogenic microbes, help in the repair and growth of skin cells, maintain skin elasticity and suppleness, slow the aging process and keep a youthful glow and natural radiance. Who doesn't want that?

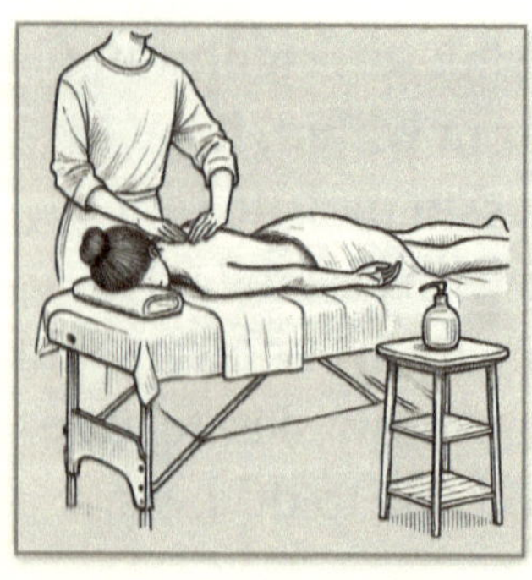

9

Eating Essentials

Now that we have understood the composition and constitution of the body along with factors that disturb its balance and learnt a few powerful correction techniques, let us shine some light on the single largest reason that is driving illness today. Looked at another way, it is the wall keeping us away from good health.

Output of robust health depends on the input of food we eat. When a holistic therapy is combined with supporting foods, the speed of return to normalcy is expedited. Right food is like fixing the leak in the boat to keep it from sinking. The

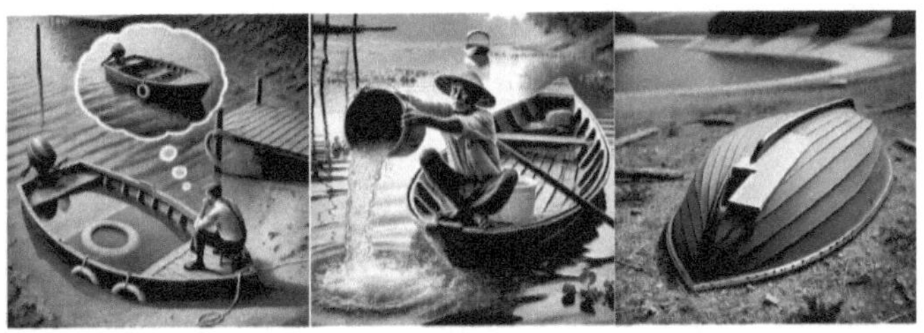

effort to keep throwing out the water (eating medicines and continuing with culprit 'foods') might work in an emergency but it is short-sighted, resource draining and enormously wasteful. <u>The leak has to be fixed</u>. Thankfully the body does a better job at fixing itself with right foods than we can do with a leaky boat. If we are looking for drug-free life and return to health what we eat *must* support all functions of our body. It is as simple as that.

Animals in their natural habitats follow this rule perfectly. Unless attacked or wounded, they are aways healthy. Animal body is also composed of the same elements as that of human body but due to their instinctual guidance, they do not eat whatever they come across. They always choose food which keeps them healthy.

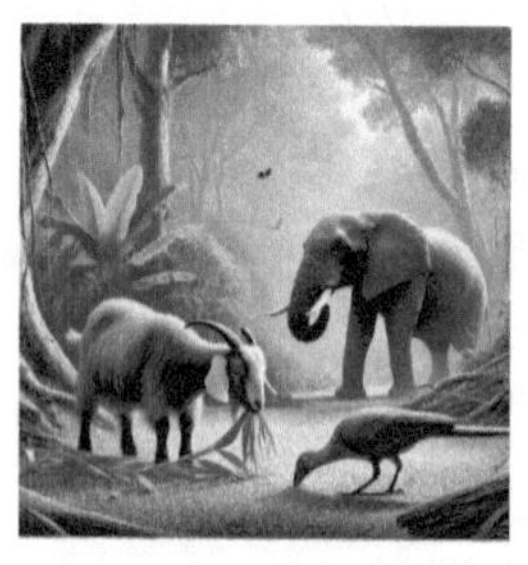

A goat eats only leaves and nothing else. A bird eats only fruits and grains. An elephant, despite its huge body, eats only plants and trees. A lion or a tiger eats flesh of other animals. It is interesting to note here because of the 'second-hand' food and not direct, plant-based food, lions and tigers (meat-eating animals) live a shorter life.

However, they are smart not to eat unnatural food that interferes with their body functions.

Animals choose provisions that nature has designed for them and their body gets all essential requirements viz. carbohydrates, fats, proteins, minerals and vitamins from food they eat. All these elements - constituents of a balanced diet- are manufactured internally by their own bodies.

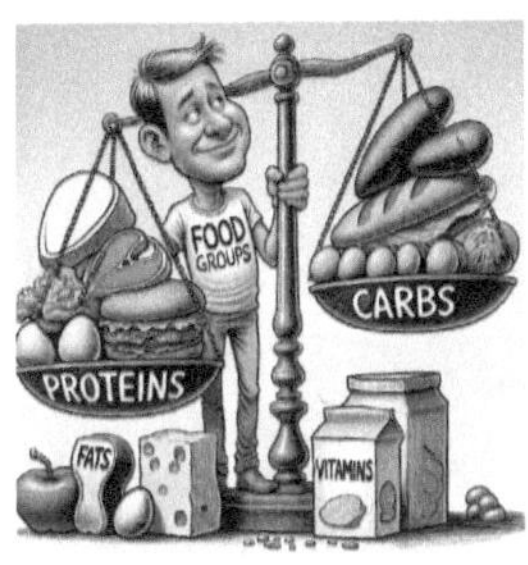

The human body has similar capacity. We can obtain the nutrients necessary for us by choosing the right foods. When we eat the variety designed by nature we do not need to seek carbohydrates, fats, proteins, minerals and vitamins separately. Like other life forms, we are assured all macro and micro nutrients without needing to weigh them.

Today the modern man has moved afar from nature. Since the distance between farm and home has increased,(s)he is being out-smarted by an industry that has learnt to trick the human mind with chemicals added into foods that masquerade as nature-made. It is therefore critical today to know what should and should not be eaten. Good health pivots on this understanding for which technical training is unnecessary. Plain old common sense suffices.

Elements of a Balanced Diet

A balanced diet, as mentioned before, is a right mix of carbohydrates, fats, proteins, vitamins and minerals.Acquainting ourselves with the different groups and knowing what they provide is helpful in making our food selection and avoid getting tricked. Let's understand each briefly.

Carbohydrates

We need carbohydrates for glucose, our primary source of energy. We get most of our carbohydrate from grains. That being so, it is vital to choose the right grains and consume it with its fiber which is the source of minerals, vitamins and beneficial microbiota.

Today paddy rice and wheat lead world-wide in consumption. Most varieties are genetically modified, grown industrially and do not provide the required

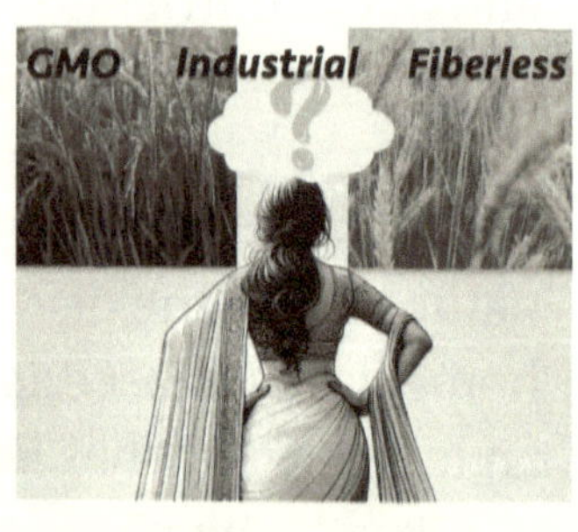

amount of fiber that our body needs. Most rice

and wheat is in fact stripped
completely of its fiber and
consumed. As long as we can
obtain whole, organically
grown grains, eat them in
correct quantities and exercise
daily, it is better to eat the variety of locally
available grains rather than go universally
with 'white' rice and wheat.

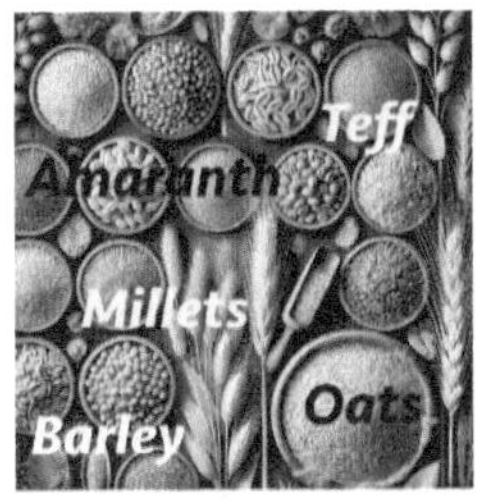

It is noteworthy that the grains with the
most fiber equipped to keep us in good health are
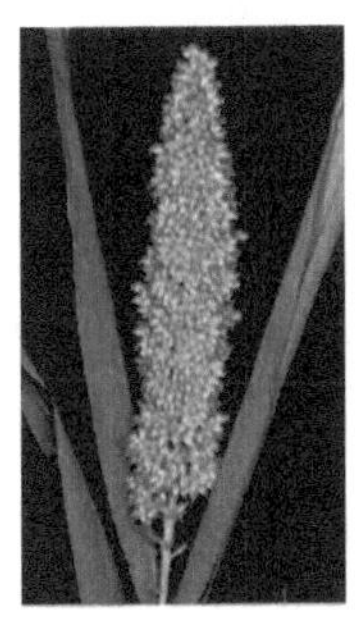
Millets. Millets use very little
resources and are capable of growing
in most geographic regions without
fertilizers or pesticides. They are
thus not burdensome on the planet.
Millets are available in plenty in India
and across the world. For that
reason, they are a good choice for
sustaining a disease-free life. As we will see in the
chapter on Millets, when we choose these grains
the whole debate on carbohydrate-free diet
becomes moot.

Protein
Proteins are essential for many functions- growth
and repair of cells, making enzymes for
biochemical reactions, immune defense, as

transport molecules for storing nutrients, and as a supplementary energy source.

Today protein is increasingly associated with

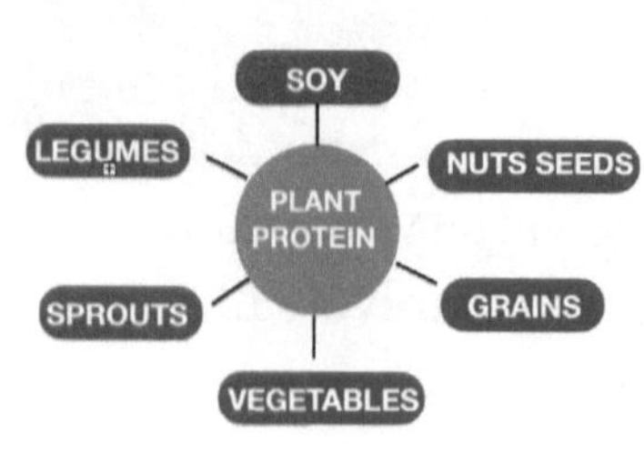

meat but for most of human history, plants have been a source of proteins. We can in fact meet all our protein requirements by eating a variety of legumes -lentils & beans, nuts (almond, pistachios, walnuts), seeds (chia, pumpkin, sunflower, *sabja*, flax, quinoa), soy (soy milk, tofu, edamame, tempeh), sprouts (micro-greens, mung, fenugreek), all <u>whole,</u> organic, non-gmo grains (millets, teff, oat, buckwheat, amaranth, wheat and rice). Vegetables too have small amounts of protein. Prominent being broccoli, asparagus, brussel sprouts, mushrooms, potatoes with skin, avocado and more.

All of these provide not just sufficient amount of protein but are a better choice for health. All we need to do is pick a whole grain and change with season the mix of other protein sources in every meal.

Our enzymes are optimized for breaking down plant-based protein and synthesize it according to our body's needs. Plant proteins have none to very little fat - about 20-26%. We are also well advised to avoid animal protein for environmental and ethical reasons that we can no longer ignore. Plant-based protein production requires fewer resources (land, water, and energy) and results in lower greenhouse gas emissions. Plant-based diets support sustainable farming practices and can help reduce the strain on the environment caused by intensive animal farming.

Resource Use & Impact

Animal farming often relies heavily on steroids and antibiotics, contributing to the global issue of antibiotic resistance and hormonal imbalance in humans. The inhumane use of steroids in animal farming pass on via meat and milk to humans and disturb the endocrine balance. In addition, there is higher chance of harmful viruses entering our bodies when we support animal farming.

Furthermore, there are economic benefits to choosing plant-based foods. Apart from a wide and delicious variety in which we can cook them, plant-based proteins are more affordable and a cost-effective choice for many people.

An important fact to note is as long as there is <u>access to locally grown diversity</u> of food, we do not see sickness due to low protein intake. Most diseases today are not on account of less but due to *over*-consumption of protein, especially animal meat.

Plant-based proteins are rich in essential nutrients like *fiber*, *vitamins*, *minerals*, *phytonutrients* and *antioxidants*, which are often 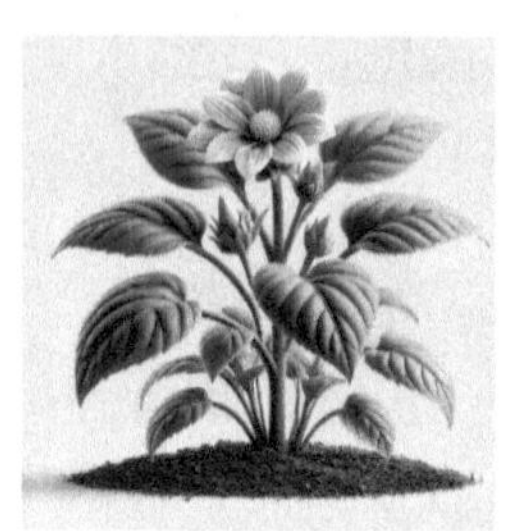 lacking in animal-based proteins. We can ensure sufficient intake of protein without getting into obsessive calculations by eating a variety of nutrient-rich plants that contain all essential amino acids. Eaten in balanced amounts, we can prevent chronic conditions including kidney diseases, type 2 diabetes, hypertension and cancer.

Fats
Good fats play several vital roles in the body. Fats provide concentrated energy to us and are essential for the absorption of fat-soluble

vitamins (A, D, E, and K). Fats are a crucial component of cell lining and help to maintain their structure and function while protecting them against physical shock and injury. They insulate the body and maintain body temperature. Essential fatty acids, such as omega-3 and omega-6, are critical for brain function and support cognitive health and mood regulation. Fats contribute to the feeling of fullness and satiety after meals, helping to regulate appetite and food intake. They also enhance the flavor and texture of foods, making meals more enjoyable. Fats play a role in various metabolic processes, including the synthesis of cholesterol and the regulation of blood sugar levels.

FATS
Protect
Satiate
Insulate
& Affect-
Mood
Brain-Health
Taste
Cholesterol
Blood-Sugar

Refined Oil

Denatured

With so many crucial roles, we cannot eliminate fat from our plate. However, for overall health and proper functioning we have to choose <u>good quality</u> fats like butter, ghee and bull-driven *ghani* oils and eat them in <u>amounts commensurate with our levels of activity</u>.

Refined oils, a product of industrialization, are highly processed oils extracted from seeds using chemicals, high temperature and pressure that denature the oils and make them harmful for our body. They are reason for disease. The age-old

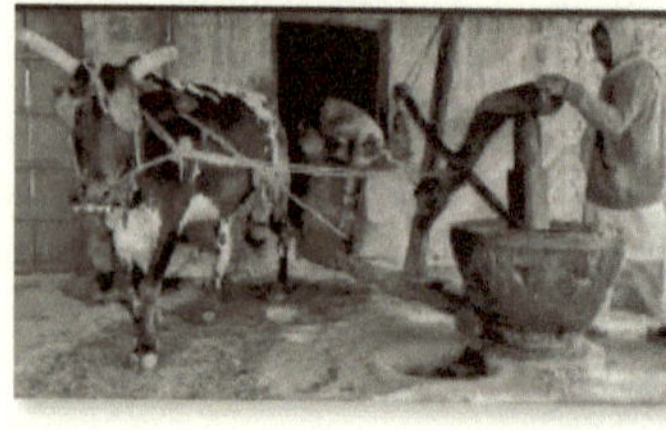

technique of cold-pressing oils at constant, low pressure using bulls provides the best quality oils that our body thrives on. ***Ghani*** and cold-pressed oils can be made from groundnuts, sesame seeds, coconuts, safflower, mustard and other seeds.

While consuming oils we need to take care to avoid oils stored in plastic containers and packets. Plastic nano-particles dissolve into oils easily and can stick to walls of our small intestine after we consume them through food. With

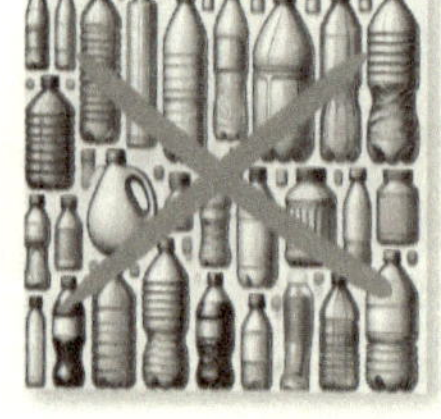

time, our intestines slowly lose the ability to assimilate nutrients from food we consume. Drinking structured water, as mentioned in

Chapter 4, helps eliminate plastic nano particles from the body.

The amount of oil to use can also vary depending on the recipe, cooking method, and individual 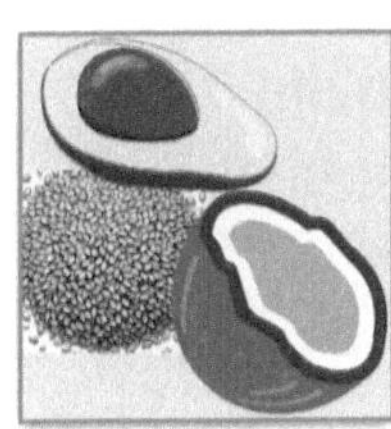 dietary needs. In general, a couple of tablespoons of oil is enough for meal preparation for four people. Sometimes the oil can be skipped entirely and whole foods with good fats like sesame seeds, shredded coconut or avocado where available, can be taken with cooked food or salads.

By being mindful of the fats we choose, we can enjoy strength and vitality into old age and be entirely free of heart conditions commonly linked to fats.

Vegetables & Fruits
Every season nature offers a feast for the senses and a powerhouse of nutrition. Each fruit and vegetable contributes to health and vitality.

To maximize the benefits from fruits, one or two types should be eaten alone either before breakfast or as a snack between meals.

Vegetables on the other hand are a perfect complement to the carbohydrate and protein on our meal plates. They are critical to boosting our health with their variety in color, taste and power. The vibrant orange of carrots bursts with beta-carotene to bolster our vision, the deep green of spinach is rich in iron and folate to fortify our blood and support cellular health.

Every vegetable delivers a vital mix of vitamins, minerals and phytonutrients. All we need to do is cook them gently with beneficial herbs and spices in good quality fats adding taste and flavor.

Industrial agriculture and growth in storage technology is spawning a culture of unseasonal consumption. It is best to choose locally available, seasonal fruits and vegetables because they are purposefully designed by nature to have specific balancing effects as per season and geography. For example high water content of cucumber and watermelon keeps us hydrated in the summer. The lycopene in watermelon also protects against sun damage. High in fiber and antioxidants, apples support digestive health and help boost the immune system as flu season begins. Rich in vitamins A and C, sweet potatoes help boost the immune system and provide a steady source of energy during cold months.

Eating foods from cold storage and out-of-season goes against Nature's laws and carries detrimental effects on health. Enjoying seasonal food on the other hand not only ensures the freshest and most nutrient-dense produce but also aligns with the body's natural needs, providing what we require to thrive throughout the year.

Vitamins & Minerals

Nature grows shapely, colorful food with each shape and hue signaling a treasure trove of vitamins and minerals. That is how life has sustained on this planet. Each life-form is tied in a symbiotic relationship to other life forms. This dependency has assured growth and suitable nourishment of all life, including humans.

Our Symbiosis with Plants

Vitamins and minerals is added separately here as a constituent of a balanced diet only to highlight the importance of obtaining them from vegetables and fruits. Ever since the scientific discovery and naming of vitamins and minerals, we have come to appreciate the many protective and physiological functions they aid; their significance in energy metabolism, DNA repair and as catalysts for numerous bio-chemical reactions needed to maintain proper body functioning.

Vitamins are classified based on their solubility, which affects how they are absorbed, transported, stored, and excreted by the body. Some vitamins like the B & C are water soluble which means they are not stored in large amounts in the body and are easily

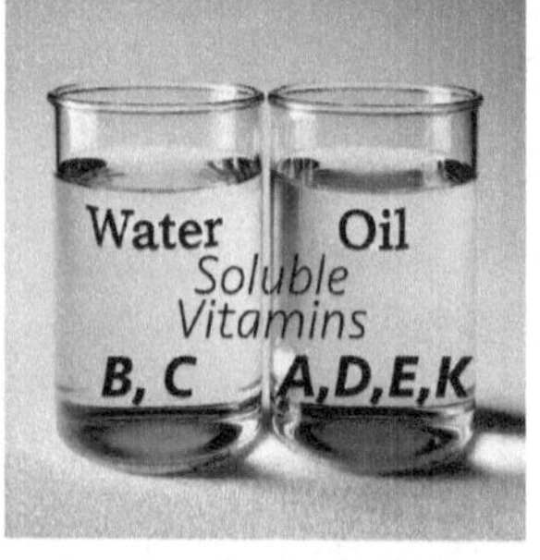

excreted in urine. They therefore need to be consumed regularly. Fat soluble vitamins are Vit A, D, E and K. Because they dissolve in fats and oils they can be stored in the body's fatty tissues and liver. They do not need to be consumed as frequently as water-soluble vitamins.

Minerals: Phosphorous, magnesium, potassium, calcium, iron, selenium, boron, zinc, copper, manganese, and, sodium (salt) are some of the important minerals required by the body. We need them for their structural role (calcium, phosphorus, magnesium), to maintain fluid and electrolyte balance (sodium, chloride, potassium), to transport oxygen (iron), for their enzyme function (zinc, copper, manganese), nerve signaling and muscle function (calcium, potassium) and proper immune health (zinc, selenium).

Where to Get Them?

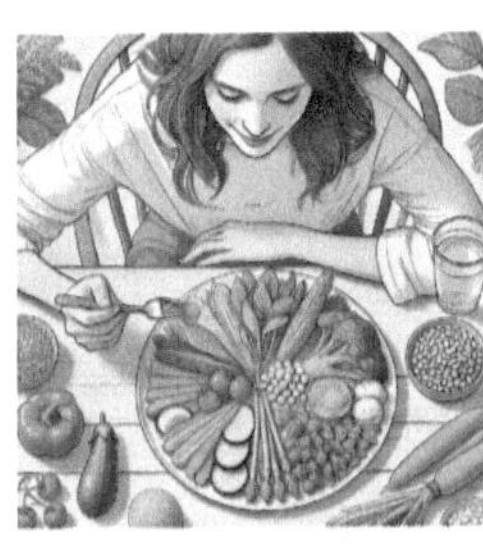

The best way to ensure adequate vitamin and mineral supply in the body is to do what holistic health sciences have been advising for centuries - eat a balanced, seasonal and local diet making sure to include a wide range of foods (not just your favorites) with focus on whole foods. Prior to the discovery of vitamins and minerals we were getting these key nutritive elements by simply eating this way.

Whole, unprocessed foods are nutrient-dense choices. They also function as probiotics as well as prebiotics, supporting growth of critical microbes in the body. Beneficial microbes play a variety of roles including manufacturing vitamins and minerals and improving our overall immunity against diseases.

We need to discriminate between food sources of key vitamins and minerals. Sometimes industries self-serving their agendas spread misinformation. For example, it is a myth perpetuated by the dairy industry that milk is the best source of calcium. There is a better way of getting natural calcium that also gives more calcium than is found in milk. One gram of calcium is present in every 100 grams of sesame seeds. Eating two sesame *laddus* of 2 inch diameter per week or chewing a handful of roasted sesame seeds daily will give the required, fully absorbable calcium to strengthen our bones. Similarly, milk made from finger millet is also a rich source of calcium.

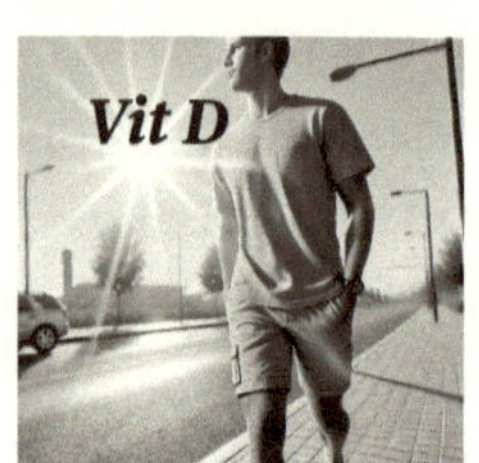

There is one Vitamin that comes from outside food- Vitamin D. To get it for free, we simply need to allow our body to make it by harnessing the free gift of sunshine. Exposing the skin to sunlight is all it takes to obtain this vitamin naturally.

Growing Vitamins & Minerals

In order to ensure there is availability of health-promoting, nutrient dense food we have to care for plants- our food- and ensure we have healthy, nutrient-rich, organic soils available to grow them fertilizers depletes the soil and kills microbial life responsible in large part for maintaining soil fertility.

Rich microbial diversity in soil is the source of taste, color and nutrition in the produce we eat. Organic farming practiced for centuries was the default way of farming and we as consumers need to push for it so it can replace the practice of industrial agriculture which has grown only in the last hundred years or so to promote sales of chemical industry.

Supplements

Vitamin shots, pills and supplements are expensive yet poor substitutes to nature's 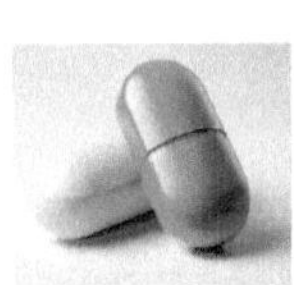 nutrition. Getting vitamins and minerals from pills is a recent development and a sign of regression than progress. While it might have a place in some situations, its growth is a reflection of our failure in applying right farming practices.

Extracting Nutrients from Whole Foods

Growth of supplement industry and packing vitamins and minerals in pills is a consequence of

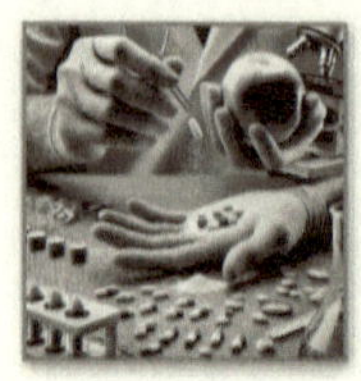 many factors. With extraction technology developing at a rapid pace, many forces are compelled to monetize discovery of each nutrient found in nature. Environmental degradation, erosion of soil fertility, growth in industrial techniques of farming and consequent fall in the quality of food become reasons to justify extraction of nutrients or worse substituting them with synthetic or lab manufactured versions.

However, for sustainability it just makes more sense to focus on restoring soil fertility and simply eat the food directly. Without fertile soil we endanger future life itself and the extraction will be a short-lived venture. If it is manufactured from chemicals then in all probability it will fail to be absorbed by the body to receive any benefit.

Nature packs many nutrients in plants that work synergistically. Just because we have discovered one nutrient and understand how it helps the body does not necessarily mean extracting and having it in high doses will yield results similar to having the whole food.

Our body is best served if we savor the bounties of nature and enjoy it straight from fertile farms and sunshine, the enabler of all food.

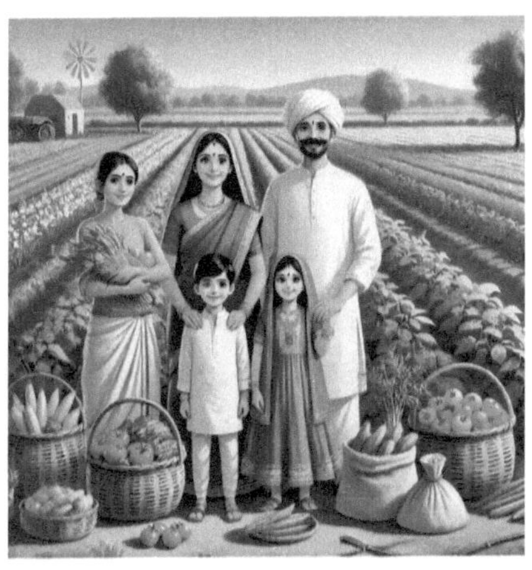

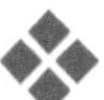

10

Food Handling

After ensuring our pantry is well stocked with all macro and micro-nutrients, we have to ascertain that we handle them correctly. This means storing and cooking them in a manner that assures the nutrition remains intact and actually goes in our body.

Microwave Oven

Microwave radiation is an accidental fall-out of research on radar technology during World War II. Although a convenience, the machine itself is built with many heavy metals and chemicals that are contaminating, non-biodegradable and pose significant health-risks. Disposing it at the end of its life is an environmental burden.

The high intensity radiation doesn't kill pathogenic

bacteria commonly found in microwaves but it does de-nature food as it heats it. The effects of the altered food particles do not offset the seeming advantage obtained from the reduced reheating or cooking-times plus the machine harbors food-borne bacteria.

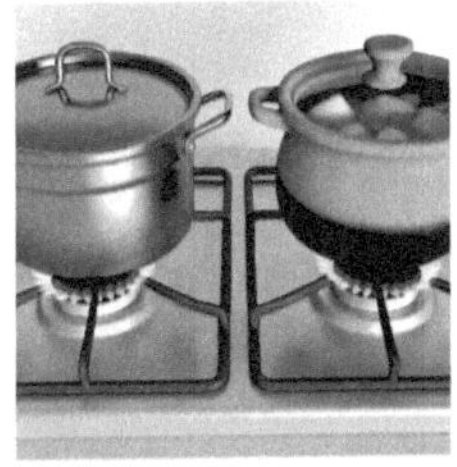 In order to preserve food nutrients it is best to cook food gently on low heat and use either the 'double-boiling method' (placing food in a steel vessel which is in turn placed in another vessel filled with hot water) or simply heating directly on low flame in a steel vessel.

Cookware

Non-stick cookware is now a common sight in homes and many cooking videos. Like microwaves, it showcases indiscreet application of accidental discoveries that have taken place in the last hundred years.

A chance finding of Teflon in 1938 led a French engineer to market the first **non-stick** fry-pan in 1954 using PTFE (polytetrafluoroethylene). The technology was allowed all over the world without adequate testing. It is well known now that polymer coatings become **toxic at high**

heats and when mixed with food cause cancer and damage to liver and all endocrine glands. They are also vulnerable to scratching by metal utensils and abrasive cleaners and degrade within 3 months. Once degraded the chemicals leach and mix with food and pose severe health hazards including risk of cancer.

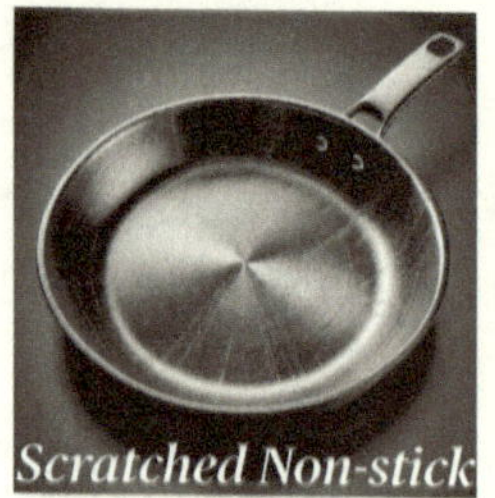

Many **air-fryers** popular today are made of non-stick materials and are best avoided.

The best vessels to cook in are clay, stainless steel, and iron. Pick skillets/*tavas*, cooking vessels and utensils made of these materials. Wood is

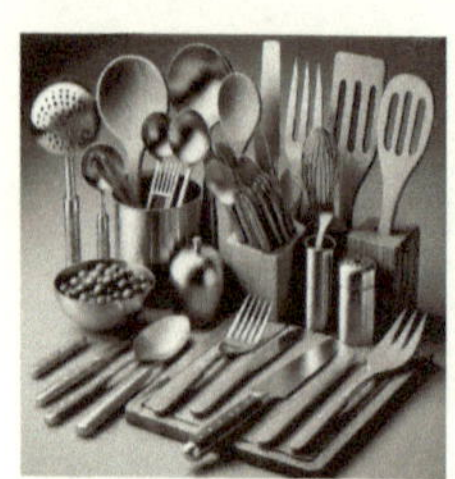

also a good choice for utensils. They last long with proper care and maintenance and are the safest choices for health- both ours and the planet's.

Manufactured & Fast Foods

Another fall-out of post World-War II, packaged and fast foods have rapidly risen since. Today we have cheap machinery to handle food- separate fiber from the whole grain, cut, chop, grind, and press vegetables and seeds. There is also easy access to low-cost chemicals that extend shelf life, color, sweeten, flavor and texturize produce. It is not surprising that manufactured food, with a little help from smart marketing, has become one of the biggest industries today.

Most packaged foods are typically made of white flour (*maida*), sugar, refined ingredients, preservatives and additives that are harmful to the body. The lasting damage caused by these foods affects many organs and in some cases is irreparable. Many diseases are seen to reverse when these fake foods are eliminated from our diet.

Restaurants may use produce for cooking but tend to cut costs by compromising on quality of ingredients, especially oils. Home-made food with choice of best quality ingredients leads to healthier eating habits and control over portion sizes. It also promotes financial well-being with less money spent on food and potential medical treatment. Always elect for freshly prepared food handled correctly and preferably consumed the same day.

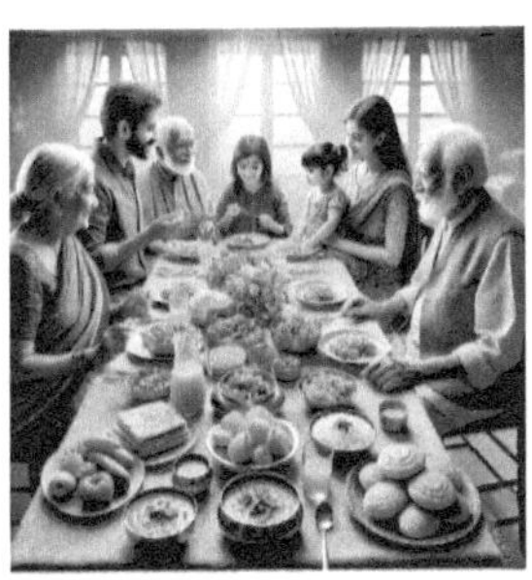

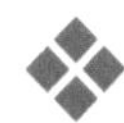

11

Millets

An exclusive chapter on Millets is added because of the potential this ancient grain holds to change the fortunes of both humankind and the planet. Very little is known or understood about Millets and its varieties, hence a brief overview of it is in place.

Millets have been around for centuries, concomitant with or perhaps longer than many other grains. Yet it is surprising that only two grains are dominating the global arena today- wheat and rice. They are subsidized and distributed in rations and doled out as aid. Even as India is promoting millets for the last few years, each of us needs to embrace and champion this humble grain. There are good reasons to do so. Millets have the power to create self-sufficiency in food, globally. Let us see how.

Nature has packed huge amounts of fiber in millets. Most of us know about the following varieties of millets- finger millet, sorghum, pearl, and proso millet.

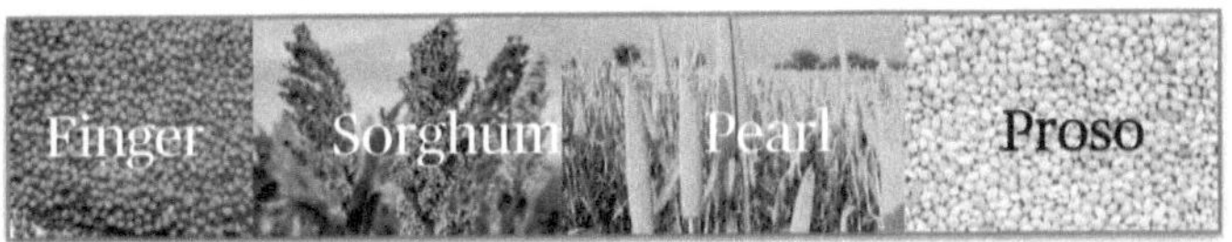

However, there are other lesser known varieties that have fiber in far greater amounts than in the above So much so that when cooked and consumed, the amount of fiber in them can control the release of carbohydrate and in turn of glucose in the blood. With these special varieties- called Small Millets- _no_ spike of sugar levels _ever_ happens. Even when eaten in hunger-satiating quantities.

This health revolutionizing quality of the grain is completely overlooked and is the reason why today the word 'carbohydrate' is treated with much disdain and rejection. The disqualification of carbs is unwarranted considering that small millets is successful in helping reverse diabetes which we are otherwise consigned to lifelong. We simply need to substitute these good wholesome grains into our plates in place of wheat and rice which cause sugar flooding and a series of ailments usually starting with diabetes and expanding to hypertension and auto-immune conditions.

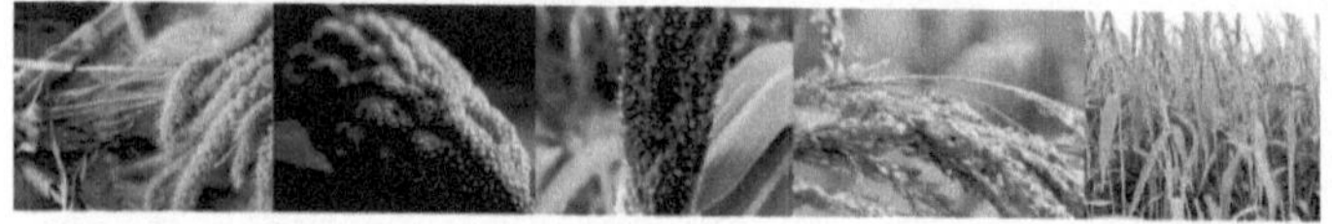

There are many varieties of small millets spread across the globe but the ones popular today are- foxtail, brown-top, little, barnyard and kodo. Eating small millets not just reconnects us with our heritage but spearheads smart resource conservation solutions that ensure continued nutritional and resource availability for the future.

Our health is intricately tied to the health of the planet. When we choose to eat wheat and rice we approve deforestation. Denuding more forests is pushing us towards climate crisis. Just as disorders in our body exhibit symptoms, changed weather patterns- droughts, high temperature and wild-fires - are symptoms of imbalance in the natural world. Wheat and rice are also the most genetically modified grains today with many ancient varieties out of existence for growing purposes.

Nature has designed millets to grow readily in varied weather conditions with very limited water and zero need for fertilizers and pesticides. There is no need to cut forests. Growing millets also populates the soil with beneficial microorganisms that help sequester carbon and restore soil fertility in a short time. Increasing soil fertility means readily available, completely absorbable nutrition for us.

That is why small millets are both a viable, efficient and elegant way out of human health crisis and equally advantageous for resolving problems that ail the planet.

Cooking Millets is easy. Simply substitute them in place of wheat and rice. A variety of dishes can be made with Millets. Fermented millets are a great source of healthful gut microbiomes and their regular consumption for a few months helps restore many imbalances.

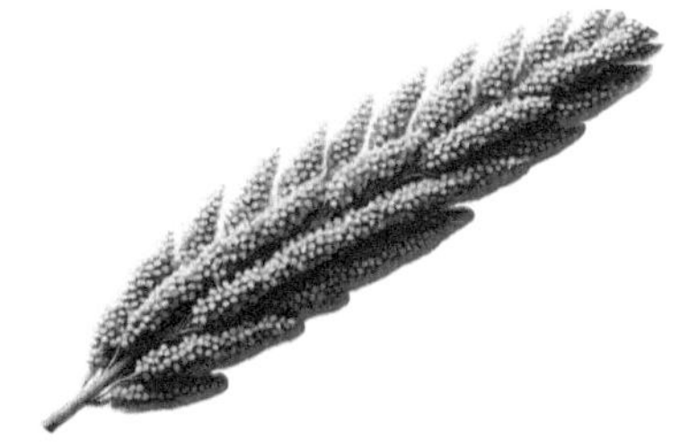

So shall we say, Millets it is!

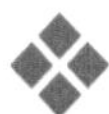

12

Invisible Friends

Our body is home to trillions of invisible microbes, including bacteria, fungi, viruses, and parasites. It is scientifically well known that we have more microbes in the body than our own cells. Most of the microorganisms reside in the large and small intestine. This diversity of flora coexists within us in a symbiotic relationship- feeding on what we eat and drink and in turn performing many important functions for us.

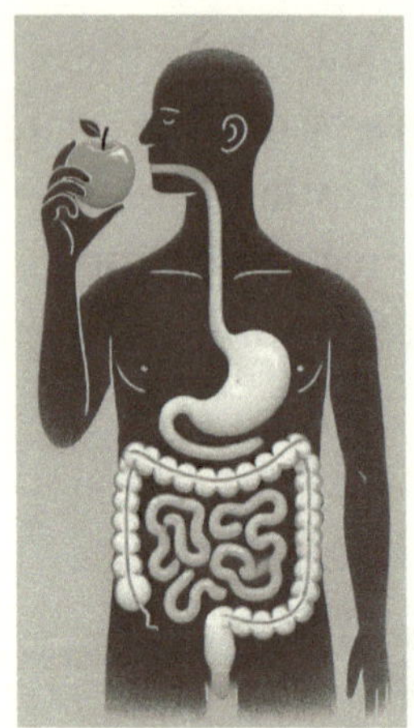

Symbiosis:
**Our food feeds
the gut flora**

The gut has the entire spectrum from health-supporting beneficial ones on the one end to potentially harmful microbes on the other. In the middle are some neutral microbiota that don't really affect us much.

Where the invisible friends come from

Good bacteria get populated in our body at the time of birth when they get passed on to us from the birth canal and through mother's milk. The food taken by the pregnant and feeding mother plays a key role in establishing good gut flora in the intestines of the developing child. Later as we grow, the composition of gut flora changes, affected by what we eat.

Where the Bad Guys come from-

A disruption or an imbalance in gut microbiota - called dysbiosis - takes place when there is faulty diet, excessive use of medicines and antibiotics. Using chemical based medicines and antibiotics kills good bacteria causing the unfriendly pathogenic micro-organisms to increase in number. This can potentially cause the immune system to become hypersensitive and trigger common GI symptoms like diarrhea, abdominal pain, and bloating.

Other factors that influence microbiota composition are environmental - what we eat and drink. Eating a variety of organic, local and seasonal produce introduces a variety of gut flora. When a diversity of micro-organisms exists in the body with a healthy balance in gut microbiome composition, the harmful pathogens get out-numbered and are rendered powerless. So the good news is we can increase good bacteria in the gut at any age.

Fermented foods like curd, buttermilk, kefir, kombucha and *ambali or* fermented porridge 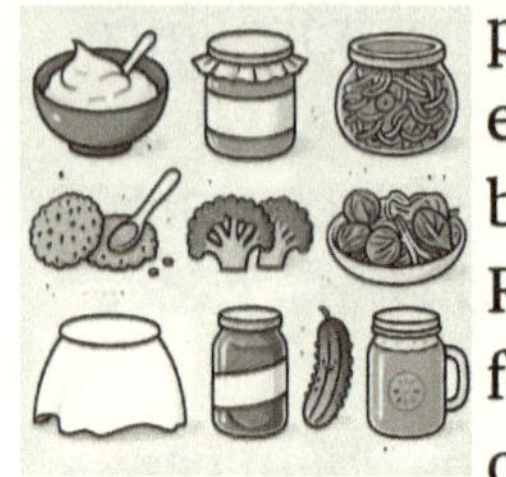 prepared from millets is an excellent way to establish beneficial bacteria in our gut. Regular consumption of these foods maintains healthy balance of gut flora. The results are *improved digestion* and nutrient absorption as well as relief from digestive disorders including bloating and constipation.

Fermented foods also *improve bio-availability of nutrients* such as vitamins and minerals in the body. This includes enhancing levels of B-Vitamins- thiamin, riboflavin, cobalamin (B-12) and amino acid tryptophan which is used by the body to make serotonin and melatonin. Serotonin is a neurotransmitter, a messenger that carries signals between cells and regulates mood, digestion, sleep and pain. Melatonin is the hormone that controls our sleep-wake cycles. Microbiome rich food is also endothermic, which means it cools the body. They *remove excess heat a common factor in allergies*. The probiotics present in fermented foods have been shown to improve allergic conditions, immunological function, and aid in disease prevention. They help to reduce inflammation in the body, which is a crucial element in the development of chronic diseases.

Cultures across the globe have included fermented foods in their culinary traditions for reasons outlined above. The tasks performed by microbes nurtured in our digestive tract by eating a diverse range of locally available, seasonal, foods along with fermented foods is key to our well being. We can easily attain and maintain optimum health by choosing only good microbiome promoting foods.

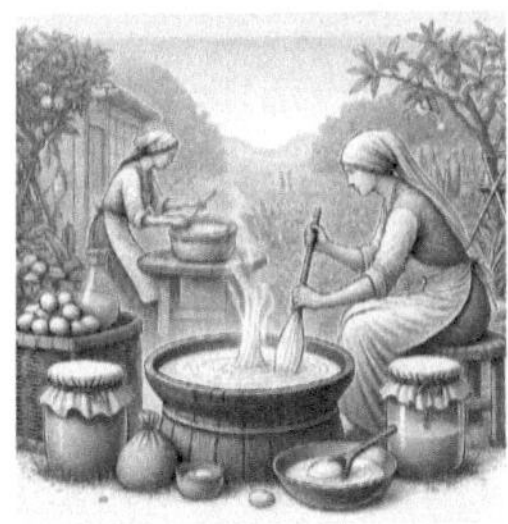

13

Kitchen Pharmacy

For centuries, common spices that grace Indian kitchens have held a revered status not just for their culinary magic, but also for their remarkable medicinal properties. Almost all share the traits of being anti-inflammatory, anti-microbial, anti-oxidant and detoxing. They

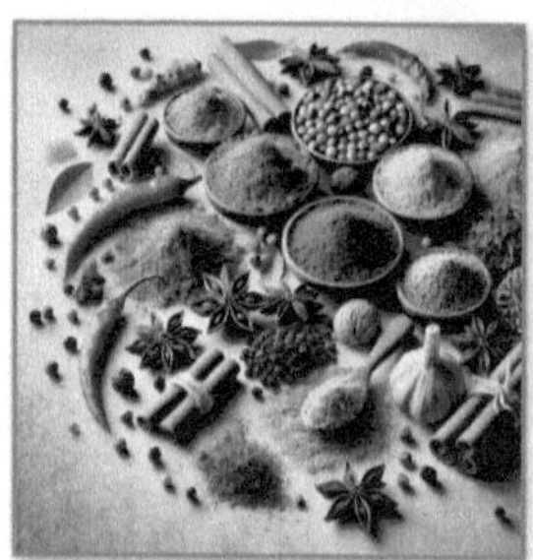

all support digestion in some way and modern science is unveiling the power of these age-old ingredients by and by, revealing their capacity to heal and nurture the body.

Embracing these spices isn't just about adding flavor to dishes; it's about unlocking a time-tested treasure trove of wellness that has been cherished for generations. Let us re-ignite the tradition of harnessing the restorative power of nature right in our own kitchen by stocking up on these wonders.

Turmeric contains a compound called *curcumin* which gives it anti-oxidant and anti-inflammatory properties. It fights common cold, boosts immunity, is both antiseptic and antimicrobial and also acts as a potent pain-relief agent.

How to Use: *For cuts and wounds* on the body, a thick <u>paste</u> of turmeric with coconut oil can be applied for quick relief. *Boost immunity & fight common cold* by drinking a <u>decoction</u> made of ginger, pepper, and turmeric.

It is best to take whole turmeric versus extracts since there are other compounds yet undiscovered that work synergistically to achieve their intended effects.

Ginger is flavorful both fresh and dry and has anti-inflammatory, anti-viral and analgesic properties.

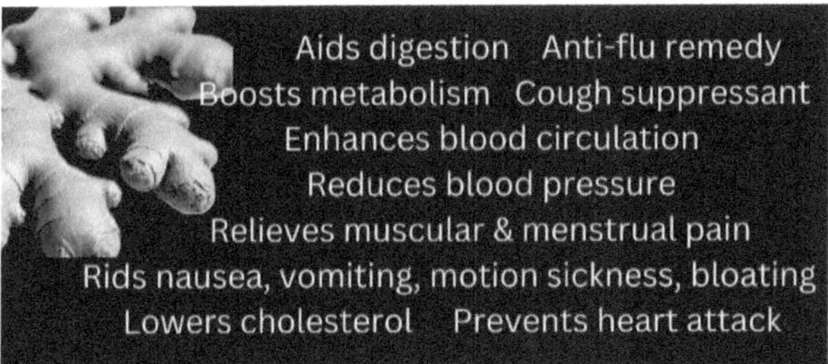

Dry ginger powder taken during initial stages of a viral infection, can ward off full blown viral illness. Just take a whiff of a few particles of dry ginger placed on the tip of a finger.

How to Use: 1. Just chew a small piece of ginger root after meals or when feeling uncomfortable. 2. As a decoction. 3. Ginger juice with honey.

Garlic has a sulphur compound called *allicin* that 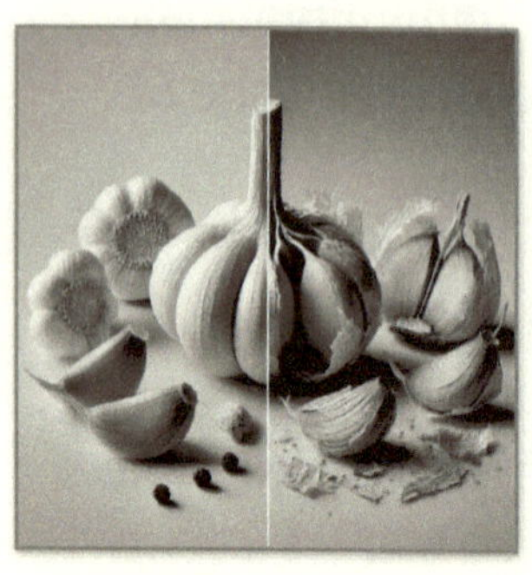 makes it medicinal. It is nature's anti-biotic and can be taken after crushing 1 clove garlic and exposing it to air for 5-10 minutes. This activates an enzyme called allinase that produces allicin. Taken continuously for 2 or 3 weeks in this way helps to get rid of undesirable microbes in the body with all the friendly ones left intact.

Allicin is also known to be anticancer, anti-inflammatory, antioxidant, and cardio-protective. It helps in deworming, detoxifying the body and also bone strength. Garlic regulates HDL cholesterol and blood pressure.
How to Use: Crush a clove and expose to air for 5-10 minutes then swallow with water. Garlic paste

applied on a painful area helps reduce inflammation and pain. It is used in many cuisines for its desirable flavor and crushing and adding it to the food is the way to use it for flavor.

Black Pepper increases the body's nutrient absorption capacity. It is commonly added to turmeric, even almond powder. It also improves the process of breaking down fat cells to produce heat which 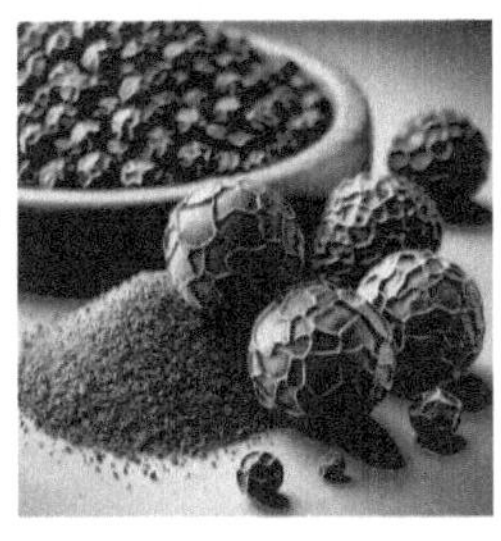 increases metabolism.Black pepper keeps the body warm, fights infections and protects against inflammation.

How to Use: Consume whole or add crushed black pepper to food, hot water or tea. One gram black pepper taken with honey helps in respiratory tract diseases. Taken with ghee it stokes appetite. *Trikatu* is an equal combination of black pepper, dried ginger powder and *pippali* (long black pepper) powder and beneficial in respiratory, hiccups, low digestive fire and catarrh conditions.

White pepper is made by taking out the black outer layer and is less heating.

Ajwain/Carom Seed is a powerhouse spice in the kitchen boasting many medicinal properties including anti-inflammatory and anthelmintic (kill parasites). These tiny seeds play a pivotal

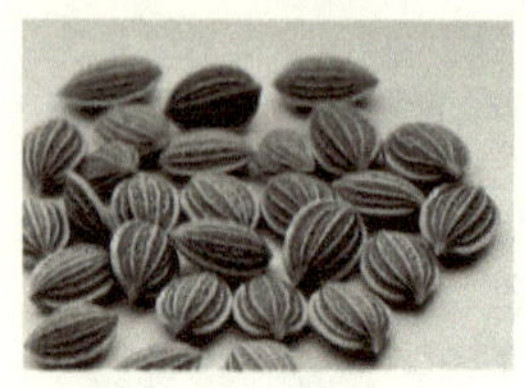

role in maintaining digestive health, alleviating all kinds of abdominal discomfort - stomach pain or burning sensation- stemming from indigestion or other factors. Being pungent, they also help stimulate the appetite and maintain robust metabolism.

Add them to oil while cooking for flavor and digestive help. Wash store-bought *ajwain* seeds and dry completely for storage and easy use.

How to Use: Simply swallow, better chew, a teaspoon after meals. In case of bloating, heaviness or flatulence after meals mix ajwain and baking soda in 3: 2 ratio and swallow with a little warm water. They can also be chewed mixed with little palm jaggery. Expectorant properties of ajwain help in clearing mucus from the respiratory tract to rid foul smell and relieve respiratory issues. It can be taken wrapped in a betel leaf and chewed well to alleviate dry cough. The juice of leaves of ajwain plant get rid of parasitic worms. It can be soaked in water overnight and consumed in the morning as ajwain water or boiled into a decoction. The boiled water can also be applied on insect bites to relief sting and help heal the skin. The decoction water can also be applied as a compress on skin to relieve itching. Used as a poultice it works as an analgesic to relieve pain due to arthritis, rheumatism and colic. It also helps in easing menstrual cramps and discomfort. Brushing with well roasted and powdered carom seeds mixed with rock salt helps maintain healthy teeth and oral cavity.

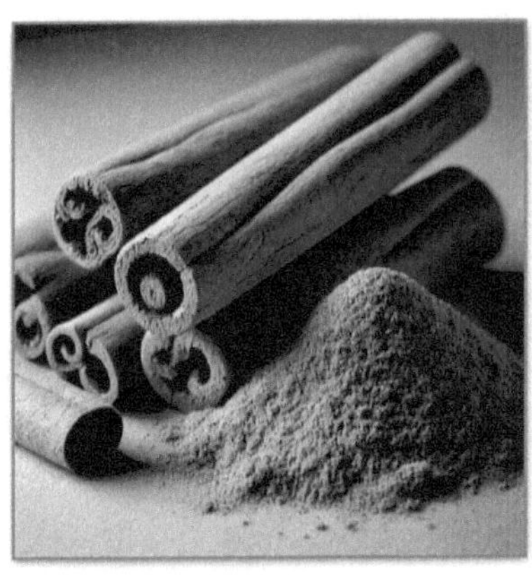

Cinnamon is a versatile spice and is sweet, pungent and fragrant at the same time. It calms both *Vata* and *Pitta dosha* used medicinally and as a herb in food. It can be used to make both sweet and savory dishes.

How to Use: Add half a teaspoon of cinnamon powder to your morning whole grain cereal, baked bread or smoothie to help regulate blood sugar levels and benefit from its antioxidant properties. Drink cinnamon tea on an empty stomach to help reduce cholesterol, manage weight, boost metabolism and reduce sweet and thirst cravings. It reduces inflammation of the mucous membranes of the mouth and is useful added to do-it-yourself (DIY) tooth-powder. Cinnamon decoction is also helpful in cold, flu and relieves sinus congestion. It reduces bloating, and alleviates gas and hence a digestive aid as well. It is also a solution to joint pains. Use it as water, tea, powder, aroma oil and mixed in with other herbs.

Asafoetida or *hing* is a gum resin taken from roots of Ferula plants. It is a digestive aid and stimulates the secretion of digestive enzymes while also relieving gas, bloating, and indigestion. It is effective in treating abdominal spasms, menstrual cramps and colic.

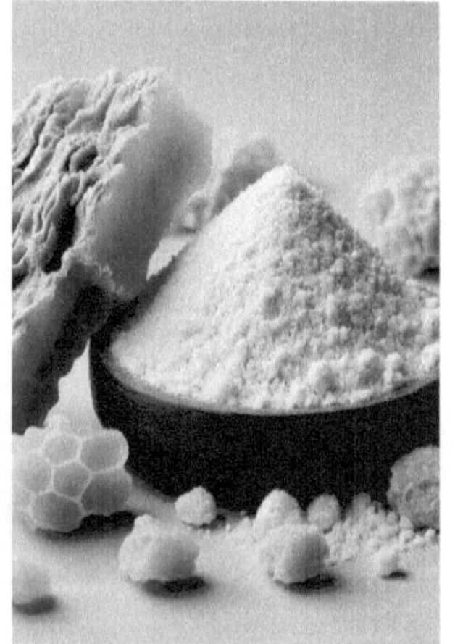

Hing has also been traditionally used for the treatment of diseases such as whooping cough, asthma, ulcer, epilepsy, stomach ache, bronchitis, intestinal parasites, and influenza.

How to Use: It can be mixed with water and put in the navel of infants to relieve pain. It can also be mixed with warm mustard oil and massaged onto the abdomen to relieve stomach cramps. A small pinch of hing can be added to oil when cooking to enhance flavor and aid digestion. For respiratory issues, *hing* can be mixed with warm water and inhaled as steam to help clear mucus and relieve congestion.

Hing is used in small amounts as it has a strong taste and potent effects. Excessive use can cause digestive upset. As with all spices, store *hing* in an airtight container in a cool, dry place away from direct sunlight.

Black Salt also called *kala namak* improves digestion by stimulating production of bile in the liver, which helps in breaking down food and absorbing nutrients more effectively. It tastes less salty but is rich in minerals like iron, calcium and magnesium which help in maintaining electrolyte balance in the body. Because it is alkaline it neutralizes stomach acid and reduces symptoms of acid reflux and heartburn and alleviates acidity. It also acts as a laxative.

How to Use: Just sprinkle a little on fruits, cooked food, salads and in lemon or plain water.

Rock Salt or *Sendha Namak,* like black salt also improves digestion and maintains electrolyte balance. It is a good remedy for digestive problems such as constipation, heartburn, bloating, and stomach pain. It is full of minerals and vitamins, promotes bowel movements and 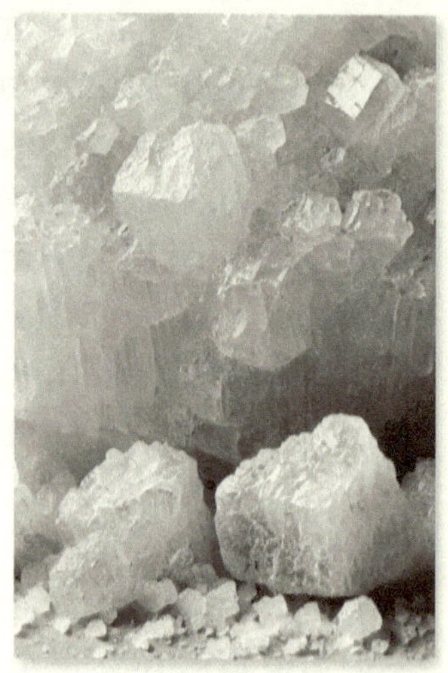 helps to clean toxins from intestines. Like ajwain and in combination with it, rock salt helps to improve loss of appetite.

How to Use: Gargling with rock salt water can help soothe a sore throat and reduce throat infections. Dissolve a pinch of rock salt in water with sugar and lemon to create an oral rehydration solution for preventing dehydration. Use rock salt in bathwater or create a paste with water and apply it to the skin to treat various skin conditions. Dissolve rock salt in warm water and soak your feet to relieve tired and achy feet, reduce swelling, and treat fungal infections. Sprinkle on salads and add to lemon juice.

Cardamom There are two types of cardamom-green and black which is relatively larger in size. The green cardamom is lighter and relatively cooling while black cardamom has a greater heating effect. Being anti-inflammatory both aid in respiratory tract problems. Green cardamom calms aggravated *vata dosa* and helps allay

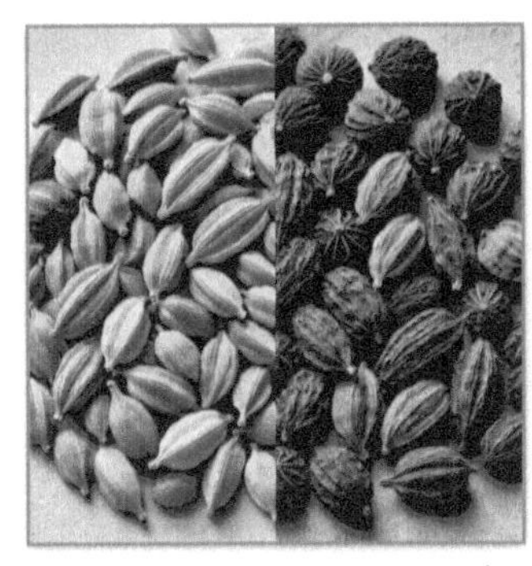

burning sensation in hemorrhoids and urinary tract issues. Black cardamom is helpful in mouth and head related issues and relieves itching. Cardamom is helpful for diabetic patients, boosts heart and liver health. It has antimicrobial properties and helps prevent ulcers.

How to Use: Chew green cardamom after meals. It is a great mouth-freshener too. Cardamom tea is very tasty and has an enjoyable aroma. Cardamom powder licked with honey and *Sitopaladi* powder is helpful in addressing mid-back problems and dryness issues.

Red Chillies contain a substance called *capsaicin* that speeds up the body's metabolism, which directly burns calories. It is also an abundant source of vitamin C which supports the immune

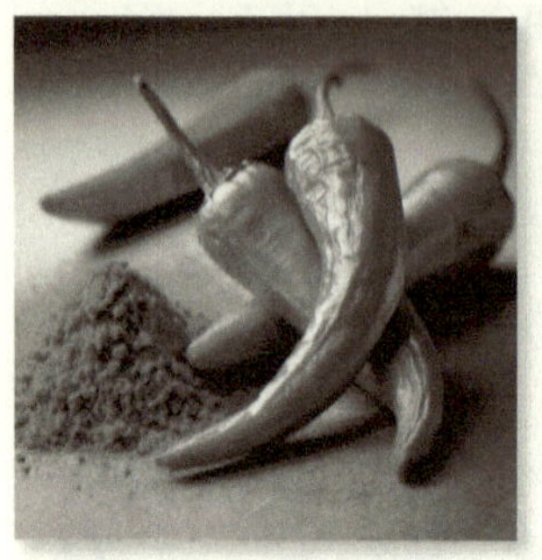

system and prevents chronic illnesses. Red chillies contains potent antioxidants that aid in unblocking arteries and blood vessels.

How to Use: Mix into cooked or raw food. It must be taken in moderation though since they are have a heating effect on the body.

Coriander/*Dhaniya* can be used for culinary pleasure as well as medicinally in several ways because of its inherent quality and compounds present- the vitamins, minerals and antioxidants.

Both coriander leaves and seeds are a good source of vitamin K which plays an important role in clotting blood. The antioxidants in coriander help remove free radicals from the body thus

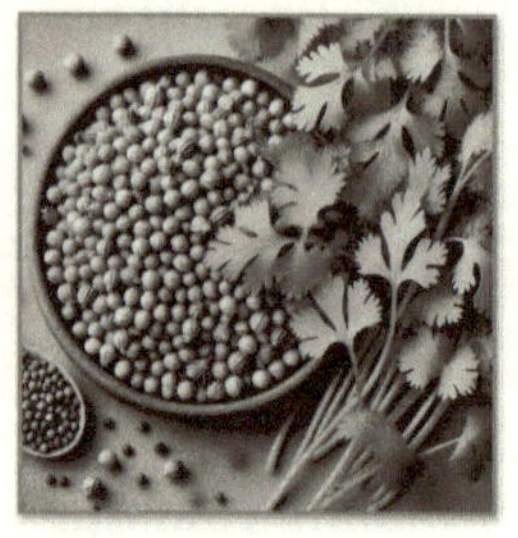

reducing the chances of cancer. Coriander seeds balance all *doshas*. They are diuretic, enhance digestion, reduce fever, help the respiratory system, remove debility and help deworm. Fresh coriander leaves or cilantro are sweet and quell increases pitta dosa and very helpful in alleviating 'heated' conditions in the body typically associated with inflammation.

How to Use: Coriander seed tea relieves indigestion, bloating, and gas. Grinding fresh coriander leaves into a paste and applying it to the skin helps reduce inflammation and soothe irritated skin. Taken as juice it helps detox and rid heavy metals from the body. They enhance the taste and visual appeal of dishes when used as a garnish.Use coriander seed infusion as a natural mouthwash to combat bad breath and promote oral health.

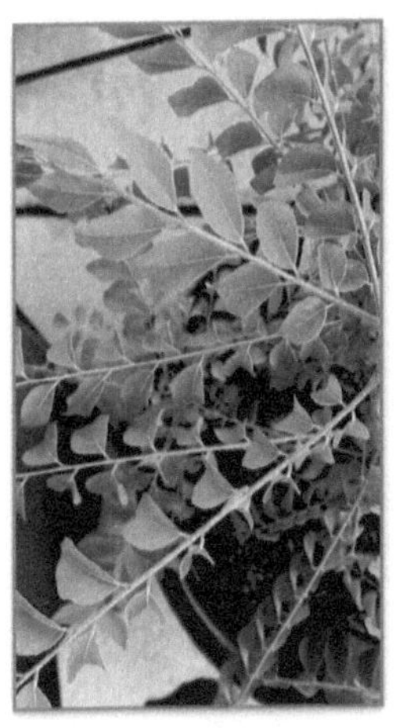

Curry Leaves are a staple in Indian cuisine. They are used in tempering to make curries, soups, dishes and to enhance flavor. Their medical benefits include reducing insulin resistance and regulating blood sugar levels. They also promote heart health because they contain a compound *rutin* and tannins that have cardio-protective properties, help lower cholesterol levels and reduce the risk of heart diseases.

How to Use: These benefits can be availed by chewing a handful leaves; using curry leaves in the form of tea by simply boiling them in water for 4-5 minutes and steeping for another 10 minutes. Dried leaves turned into powder can be sprinkled on dishes or mixed into a chutney. Curry leaves also help in reducing hair fall, treating dandruff, and promoting hair growth. Use them in oil and boil till they turn black. Strain and use the oil to massage into the scalp. Crushing a handful of curry leaves and leaving it in buttermilk for upto half hour and drinking helps increase hemoglobin. It is easy to grow curry leaf tree in the house garden or even in a pot to have ready access to it.

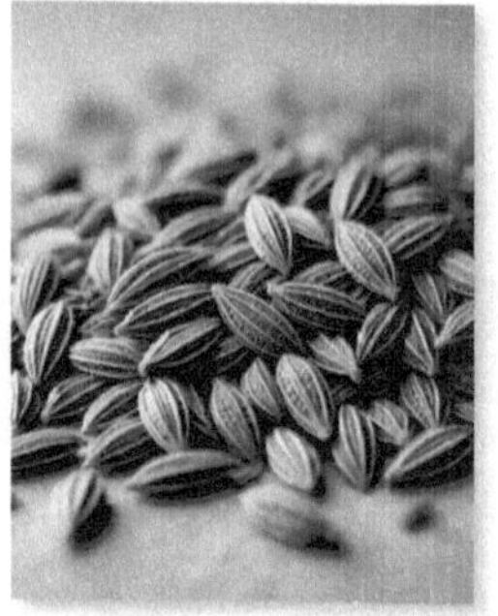

Cumin Seed/*Jeera* is an important spice that not only makes food delicious but has numerous health benefits. No spice can match the multiple benefits of cumin and its unique aroma and taste. Cumin seed have medicinal properties that can fight diabetes, epilepsy, tumors and increase immunity. They are a good source of iron and help women suffering from anaemia. Cumin seeds stimulate salivary glands thereby easing digestion process.

How to Use: It can be soaked at night in water and had in the morning as *jeera* water. It can also be used to prepare a decoction by itself or in combination with coriander and fennel seeds as a powerful digestive aid that boosts metabolism.

Black cumin seeds have greater medicinal uses. 1-2 grams of black cumin seed powder taken with warm water cures colic. Half teaspoon roasted and powdered black cumin seed added to curd and taken helps control diarrhoea and vomitting. For children honey or desi *khand* can also be added.

Fenugreek is rich in fibre, protein, chlorophyll, vitamins and minerals like iron and magnesium. Both the seed, fresh and dry leaf offer excellent health advantages and help resolve eighty types of disorders involving the air element. Fenugreek helps in correcting anemia and fatigue. The tender leaves are less bitter. As a green vegetable it reduces and regulates acidity in blood and is very beneficial for *vata* and *kapha* disorders, pregnant and lactating women. It helps in detoxing, fever, pain, depression, vomiting, cough, gout, piles, low blood pressure and to get

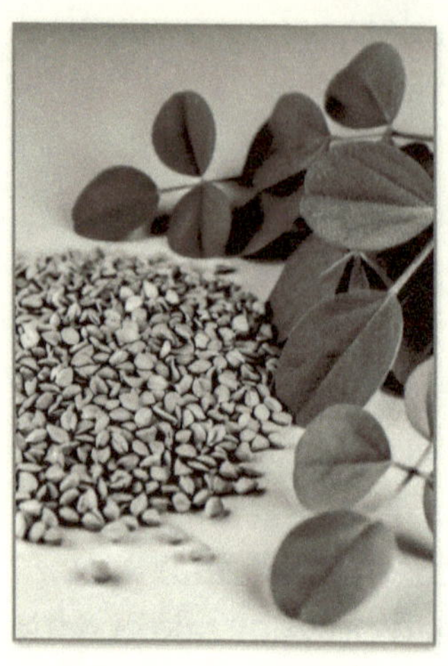

rid of worms. The seed is also used for tempering food. It aids digestion, helps blood sugar control, and reduces inflammation.

How to Use: For diabetics, drinking 100 ml of the juice every morning is very useful, In case of low blood pressure, cooked fenugreek with ginger and garam masala is helpful. For worms in children, 1-2 teaspoon of the juice taken daily is helpful. Fenugreek seeds can be soaked and sprouted for boosting its benefits. It can be taken powdered with ginger and turmeric to ease knee pain. Fenugreek also stimulates hair growth. A mask can be made with fenugreek and applied or the seeds can be boiled in water, cooled and used for hair wash. Fenugreek decoction can be made easily.

Indian Bayleaf/*Tejpatta*

Bay leaf is particularly effective in balancing the *Vata dosha*. So it is helpful in reducing gas, bloating, and other digestive issues. Bay leaf also helps in balancing *Kapha dosha* and aids in reducing congestion and clearing excess mucus from the respiratory system. *Tejpatta* is used to control diabetes due to its antioxidant and anti-inflammatory properties. It prevents the damage to pancreatic beta cells and enhances insulin secretion.

How to Use: Inhalation of steam infused with bay leaves or consuming bay leaf tea can help in relieving respiratory symptoms. Bay leaf has anti-inflammatory properties. A paste made from bay leaves can be applied topically to inflamed areas and to cuts and wounds to prevent infection. Bay leaf oil
can be used for massage. Bay leaf is used to reduce stress and anxiety. Burning bay leaves and inhaling the vapors is a traditional practice believed to help calm the mind and reduce stress.

It gives a great flavor and taste when added to food but must be used in moderation because of its heating/*pitta* enhancing effect.

Fennel (*Saunf*) is sweet tasting and commonly taken after meals to combat bad breath. However, the benefits of fennel go way beyond that. It is antispasmodic and a digestive aid and is even better if taken after roasting.

It is helpful in colic,
deworming and binding
stool. Fennel balances
vata and *kapha* dosha,
and keeps eye conditions
at bay. Fennel is used in
herbal remedies to reduce
fever and promote
sweating. When added to
the diet, it also improves
heart health, reduces
inflammation and also

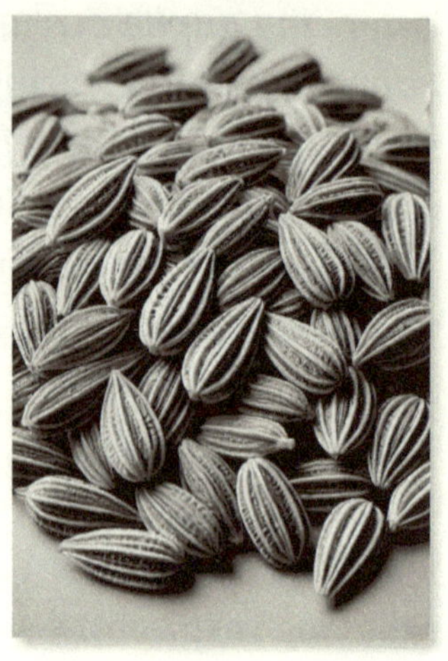

provides anti-cancer effects. Fennel is also used
to regulate menstrual cycles and alleviate
symptoms of menopause due to its
phytoestrogen content. Nursing mothers
consume fennel to increase milk production.

How to Use: Fennel seed can be chewed directly
or used to make tea or decoction. Fennel tea is
safe for infants in small doses and relieve colic
and gas pains. If there is a burning sensation
during urination, soak some fennel seeds in hot
water and drink upon cooling. An equal mix of
regular and roasted fennel seeds taken three
times a day helps alleviate sweaty palms.
Powders of fennel seed, almond powder and
black pepper help improve vision.

Nutmeg (*Jaiphal*) is also used in both sweet and savory preparations involving baking and seasoning. It has been used as medicine by

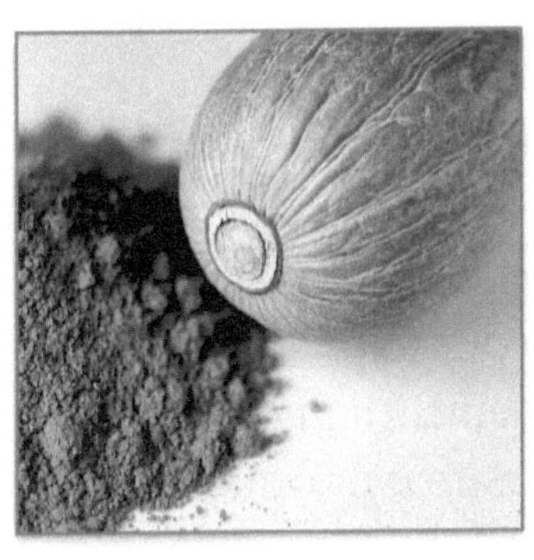

cultures across the world for centuries. It is a carminative, reducing flatulence and an appetite stimulant. Nutmeg oil is used in inflammatory conditions like arthritis to relieve pain. It enhances blood circulation to the brain and is neuroprotective but should be consumed in moderation. In some cultures, nutmeg is used as an aphrodisiac and to enhance sexual health. It also alleviates menstrual cramps and regulate menstruation. Care must be taken in using it in small amounts or under guidance for chronic issues.

How to Use: It is often made into a paste or powder and ingested. Nutmeg powder can be taken with warm milk for calming and mildly sedative effect. For respiratory ailments such as coughs and colds it is made into a tea or used as an inhalant. It can be used this way to promote sleep and reduce stress. It is applied topically, its seeds ground into a paste and applied to treat skin issues such as acne, eczema, boils, and rashes. It helps in detoxifying and rejuvenating the skin. Nutmeg is used to treat oral health issues like toothaches and bad breath. The seeds are chewed or used in concoctions for mouth rinses.

Cloves is heating but at the same time light and drying in effect. It adds flavour to food along with providing many health benefits. High in antioxidants they help regulate blood sugar and kill pathogenic bacteria. Cloves assist in digestion by lending plenty of warmth to any dish. It is also an age-old remedy to get immediate relief from tooth pain.

How to Use: Clove oil is well known for relieving toothaches and is a key ingredient in herbal tooth-powders. 1-2 cloves can be chewed or kept in the mouth. Clove decoction can be made by itself or in combination with other spices like black pepper and cardamom. It is used for tempering vegetables and lentils.

Mustard Seeds are pungent, heating and balance *Kapha* and *Vata dosha*. They are also a good source of several vitamins like Vitamin C and K, thiamin, riboflavin, vitamin B6 and folic acid. They are also a storehouse of several minerals such as copper, calcium, iron, magnesium, phosphorus, potassium, sodium, zinc, manganese and selenium. They promote warmth and circulation, alleviating cold and dryness that often accompany *Vata* imbalances.

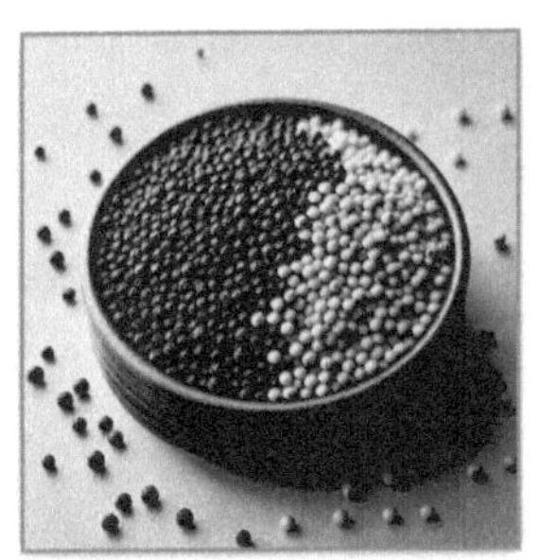

How to Use: Mustard seeds are commonly used for tempering and remove health damaging oxidants from cooking oil. In fact used as mustard oil it provides multitude benefits for strengthening the body, improving the skin, removing excess mucus, improving metabolism, and stimulating digestion. The seeds can be used to make mustard seasoning to eat with salads or cooked food.

Pickles are almost a necessary accompaniment to food, especially Indian cuisine. They bring together several spices in their making process and hence their addition here was inevitable. Controlled consumption of Indian

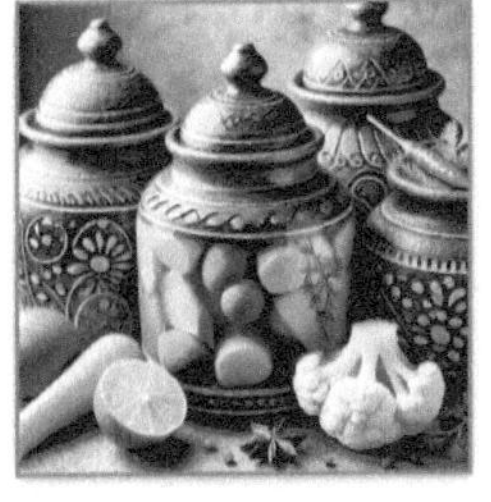

pickles adds a zing to every meal and brings with it a host of health benefits. Unfortunately, we are misled into thinking that eating pickles raises blood pressure. Prepared the right way - using the power of the sun along with high quality ingredients including *ghani* oils- pickles are full of probiotics, organic acids, and antioxidants which bolster our immune system and keeps cancer at bay.

This is the reason pickle-making is celebrated by families across India and undertaken as a social activity at special times during the year. It is in our best interest to continue the valuable cultural tradition and relish pickles as part of our daily food.

The method of preparation is important but care must also be taken to store pickles in ceramic or glass containers. Like fats and oils that easily absorb nano particles of plastic, pickles with their acids and fats also leach plastic that can enter our body and disturb its function and balance.

Healthy and tasty pickles can be made from many vegetables and fruits including lemon, mango, 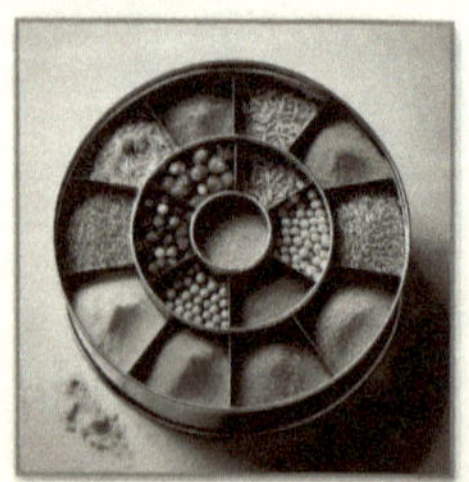 tamarind, amla (gooseberry), green leafy vegetables, tomato, chillies, cauliflower, turnip, and carrot.

14

Defining Food

It is clear that what we eat is implicated in our health. Most problems growing rapidly today can be attributed to mistaken understanding of food. Once we agree upon what food is and practice it, many problems are prevented and conditions start disappearing.

So what is food? It stands to reason that food must :-

- Maintain the key balances - glucose, hormonal and microbial- in the body. That is to say, it must not cause sugar spikes, nor interfere with proper hormone production nor kill beneficial gut flora.
- Energize and strengthen the body
- Enhance life
- Be tasty and enjoyable
- Delight and open the heart

Three Key Balances

The first aspect in understanding the term 'food' lies in appreciating the way in which we grow and process produce. We might be taking utmost care in ensuring intake of the entire spectrum of nutrition - carbs, proteins, fats, et al, but if while farming or processing, harmful chemicals are added or sprayed that cause hormonal or microbial imbalance upon consumption, then the

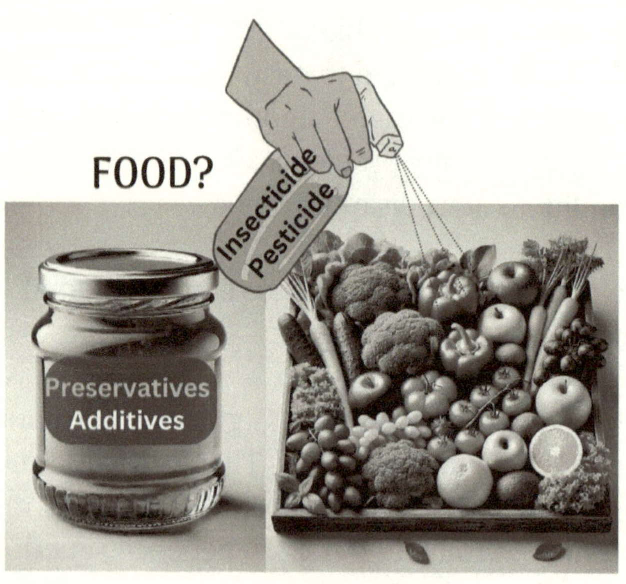

whole effort of balanced food intake becomes moot. Additionally, if we strip away key parts of produce, like fiber on grains where valuable nutrients live, we have again denied ourselves a very important control factor of good health-maintaining glucose balance.

Pleasure

Next, we must definitely choose to put on our plates foods we enjoy. It is documented in holistic practices that food eaten with pleasure brings benefits and one eaten as punishment or disdain is bereft of any goodness. Luckily, there is enough choices Nature gives to satisfy every palate's nutritive needs.

Taste

The third aspect connected to the definition of food is straightforward - its taste. While we develop preferences for certain tastes - primarily sweet, salty and sour, there are other tastes nature has designed. Ayurveda describes six tastes in food and recommends taking them daily in appropriate quantities for balance and well-being. Remember some tastes are acquired and some change with time. Keeping an open mind and knowing it brings benefits can condition the mind into accepting tastes we are not accustomed to. Each of the six taste classified in Ayurveda offers unique benefits. Here they are with examples:

- **Pungent** supports metabolism and include heating spices like black pepper, ginger, green and red chillies.

- **Salty** is needed for fluid balance. Example is obvious- sea salt, rock salt. Iodized salt is harmful and should be avoided. Natural sources of iodine are completely bio-available and should be preferred over potassium iodide, a synthetic iodine.
- **Astringent** is helpful for healing, repair and growth. All cooking oils like sesame oil, ground nut oil, safflower oil, ghee, lentils and beans are astringent. Aloe vera is also in this category.
- **Sweet** provides strength and nourishment. Clear examples are grains, jaggery of sugar cane, palm jaggery, sweet fruits, and date palm jaggery.
- **Bitter** is needed for detoxification. Examples are fenugreek seeds, bitter gourd, neem leaves, dandelion.
- **Sour**. It helps in digestion. Lemon, yogurt, amla, mango, lime, and tamarind are good examples.

The six tastes delight us in different ways. While we can have preferences for each taste, food must also bring friends and family together for community enjoyment. It is a great path to everyone's heart and helps open up people. This does not mean limiting ourselves only to salty or sweet dishes but ensuring that all the variety of tastes is present. This can be easily achieved with a combination of fruits, vegetables, grains, spices, and legumes in appetizers, meals and snacks. For example, a meal can include sweet whole grains, sour lemon pickles, salty seasoning, bitter greens, pungent spices like ginger, and astringent beans or lentils. This not only satisfies the palate but also supports overall well-being by addressing all bodily needs. Luckily we only need to eat a small amount of bitter and astringent foods.

We have already read about spices in the last chapter. They are quintessential to all cuisines, especially Indian. They all contribute in unique ways to the six tastes and more significantly, are potent remedies in themselves.

Most food we eat is cooked or eaten raw. Another form of raw food is juices.

Juices:
We write about juices here because they provide ready nutrition to the body and are good not just during convalescence but also otherwise. They support and are easily enjoyed by all ages. Although they do not have *insoluble* fiber they are not completely lacking in fiber since juices have some *soluble* fiber in them. They must be made and consumed fresh. No sugar need be added because they are naturally delicious. A wide

variety of juices can be made with seasonal vegetables and fruits. Some examples of juices are:

- Cleansing juices (ideally 8 to 9 am): Amla juice in best in winter and Bel juice in summer. Lemon juice can be taken through the year.
- Medicinal juices (on waking): Ginger, Lemon, mixed with honey.
- Other Juices for Health (4 to 5 pm):Orange, pineapple, pomegranate, coconut water, carrots, beets, apples, cucumbers, spinach, celery, and more!

Choose to have a good juicer in the house and bring your creativity to make delicious, healthful juices.

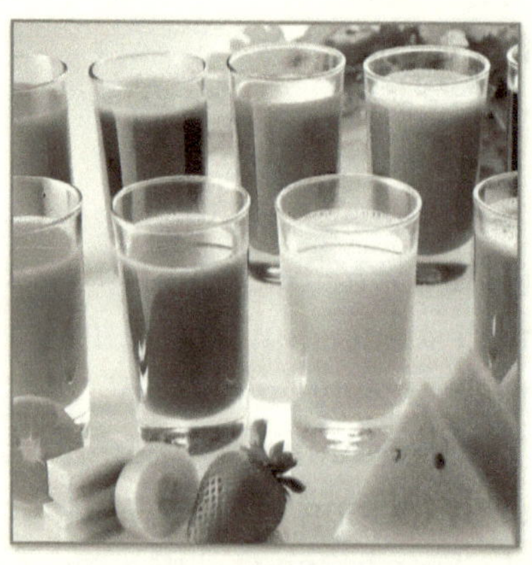

15

Home Remedies

Now that we have a basic understanding of our body, are familiar with several therapeutic techniques, and acknowledge the role of food, herbs and spices in healing, we are ready to put them all together in the event of common ailments we might face. This section connects to root causes and therapeutics discussed in preceding chapters and furnishes guidelines on how to utilize things present in our own home. There are many common ailments that inflict us throughout life and though these are not deadly, they cause a lot of misery. Let us go through some of these and check out their symptoms, causes and easy remedies.

1. COMMON COLD

This is the most common ailment and there is a joke about its remedy - if you take medicine, you will be alright within 6 days but if you do not take medicine you will be alright within a week!

First let us ascertain the root cause of this widespread affliction and understand it from the perspective of our body's constituent elements as discussed in Chapter 2.

Our body consists of about 72% water. Heat and cold have the same effect on water inside the body as they do outside. Our body also has an air-conditioning as well as a heating system with built-in thermostats. It maintains a temperature of 98.6 F (37 degrees C) in both summer and winter. The water in our body gets heated during the day due to activity and outside temperature.

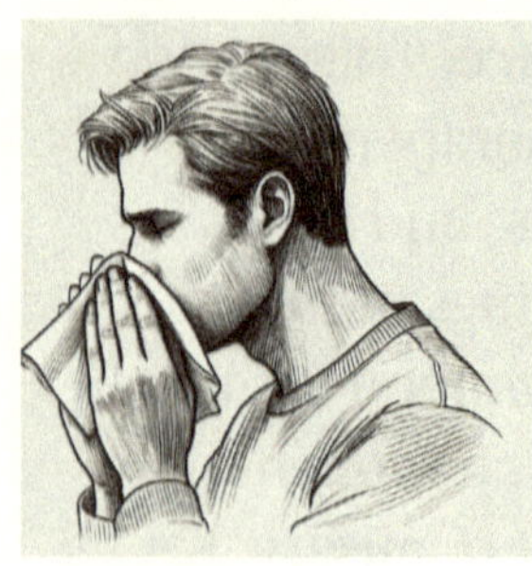

It cools down at the night creating moisture in the lungs and head. In Nature this moisture drips down as dew. In the case of our body, it is expelled by sneezing or watering of the nose in the morning.

Therefore, sneezing in the morning is a sign of good health.

However, when the sneezing and runny nose continues throughout the day and for multiple days, it is called common cold.

The heat in our body depends upon its digestive power. When the digestive system weakens, the internal temperature goes down. This reduces evaporation and causes gathering of excess water in the body. The excess water in turn reduces heat, resulting in congestion of lungs, chest and throat. When this water gets congested in the head, it causes headache. Continued cycle of excess water leads to tonsillitis, sinus trouble, bronchitis and fever.

Accumulation of water is aggravated by cold drinks, heavy food items, sour foods like curd and buttermilk and also by exposing the body to cold wind or cold temperature through air-conditioning. All these add to prolongation and aggravation of the disease.

The treatment that is helpful is one which increases heat and reduces water in the body. This is achieved in the following ways :
- Reduce intake of foods such as raw green leafy vegetables that contain too much water. This helps to control water in the body thereby speeding recovery.
- Eat warm and light foods - soups cooked with spices like black pepper, ginger, cloves, cinnamon, cardamom and cumin. They provide

heat to the body and support the digestive
system. Proper digestion is key.
- Fruits in natural form is helpful as they provide
digestive enzymes and nutrients.
- Eat gently cooked food - steamed, boiled, baked
or cooked on low heat.
- Drink lukewarm water throughout the day.
- Drink a mix of a teaspoon each of ginger juice,
lemon juice and honey on empty stomach.
- Practice *suryabhedi* pranayam to increase heat
in the body.
- If possible and necessary, undertake complete
fast for one day or eat only one meal a day.
- Steam inhalation or steam bath gives relief by
softening the tissues, loosening the deposits and
expediting cleansing.

Common Cold is no longer a malady of winter
when exposure to cold precipitates the ailment.
With <u>wrong food choices that tax the digestive
system and incorrect lifestyle that leads to
imbalance in the five elements</u>, cold (also known
as allergies now) has become very common in all
seasons. Using antibiotics is not the answer
because they do not work on viruses. Neither is
food testing & elimination of all foods as in the
case of allergies. The answer lies in eliminating
harmful chemicals, packaged foods, and
choosing produce that is grown without the use

of GMO seeds, glyphosate, synthetic fertilizers and pesticides. Lifestyle changes and natural remedies suggested above are the way to faster relief and safeguarding against continued and growing imbalance. Neurotherapy is another effective addition to dietary and lifestyle changes for allergies.

2. CONSTIPATION

Mother of all diseases, constipation is a major problem in itself but compounds trouble if left unaddressed. This makes perfect sense if one accepts that accumulation of waste is not a desirable condition anywhere - vehicle, home or in the body. Waste is meant to be cleaned out and expelled but if it continues to stay within the body or vehicle, it gives birth to more trouble.

People of all ages, including a one year-old child, can be affected by this problem. It is the root cause for many conditions like migraine, piles, hemorrhoids, fistula, fissures, peptic ulcer, colitis, chest pain, arthritis, mental illnesses, cramps in the legs, and more.

These are clear symptoms of constipation:
1. Elimination of stool does not happen daily but only once in two or three days.
2. Solidification of stools and therefore difficulty in elimination.
3. Stools in pieces, oily or foul smelling.
4. Need to sit for a long time on the toilet seat.
5. A lot of pressure needed for elimination.
6. No relief even after elimination.
7. Sleeplessness.
8. Absence of hunger.

The causes for constipation are linked to poor lifestyle choices and include:
a) No or very low intake of fibre in diet. Roughage missing in food.
b) Consuming foods like all-purpose flour/*maida* that stick to the gut lining and compromise its function.
c) Eating without hunger, overeating and inadequate chewing which does not release sufficient digestive enzymes either in the mouth or the stomach. This weakens the digestive system, creating undigested food particles and straining the elimination organs.
d) Choosing fast, fake, sugary and junk foods like ice-creams, fried foods, cold drinks, gas-producing foods that are high in additives, preservatives and lacking in nutrition and fiber.

e) Preference to animal protein that needs longer
   time to digest and sits in the system for extended
   period.
f) All intoxicants and addictive substances
   including tea, coffee, smoking that slow the
   functioning of all organs.
g) No exercise or movement which reduces blood
   supply to organs and therefore nourishment and
   leads to overall sluggishness in the body.
h) Not getting sufficient sleep and rest.
i) Stress.
j) Stopping or postponing the natural urge of
   passing stool and urine.
k) Over medication.
l) Using Western-style toilets styled for comfort
   and not designed to put the right pressure and
   provide support to the body to eliminate waste.
m) Eating in a disturbed state of mind.

The treatment for constipation is as simple as
removing all the causes responsible for it. We
have to understand that medicines do not cure
the disease. Taking laxatives increases
dependence on them and does nothing to
strengthen the body's own devices to naturally
eliminate waste. With time the efficacy of
laxatives reduces and the body is weakened even
more.

Internal remedies to help correct constipation are:

1. Avoiding low and zero fiber carbohydrates like rice and wheat and replacing them with millets which have high amounts of nutrient-rich fibre. Adding vegetables like tender bottle-gourd, ridge-gourd, and raw banana in curries is also effective.

2. Drinking a minimum of two litres water daily and at least two glasses of warm water in the morning upon waking.

3. Drinking *amla* juice which is rich in Vit C daily on empty stomach.

4. In summer, juice of Bel or pomegranate is helpful.

5. Fruits like guava which contain roughage provide good relief. Papaya removes the stickiness in intestines.

6. Bitter gourd juice and ash gourd juice helps detox and clean up the system.

7. It is helpful to eat *anjeer*/fig, *munakka*/black grape raisins, *kishmish*/golden raisins because they contain minerals that strengthen intestinal motility. They must be soaked overnight before eating empty stomach in the morning.

8. Choosing 80% of food we eat in natural form (alkaline food) like fruits, salads, sprouts and seeds and 20% in gently cooked food form.

9. Avoiding acidic, fried, fast and all packaged
   foods.
10. Chewing food well before swallowing is very
    important because the release and mixing of
    digestive enzymes starts in the mouth.

External body work for ridding constipation are
as follows:
1. Using Indian toilet or doing *Mal-asana* every day
   for 5-10 minutes after drinking water.
2. Pelvic or tub bath once a day with regular or
   warm water.
3. Cooling the intestines by applying mud or cold
   pack for 15 minutes daily in the morning.
4. Spinal bath.
5. Enema with plain water for a week to cleanse
   out the intestines completely.
6. Doing *Agnisar kriya* and *Shankaprakshalana* -
   two powerful yogic *kriyas* for strengthening the
   intestines and increasing motility.
7. Daily exercise, pranayama, and meditation is
   essential. Choose what you like from walking,
   swimming, biking, a sport or yoga asanas.
8. Sitting in *Vajrasana* for 10 minutes after meals.
9. Correct position of Solar plexus/*nabhi* because
   displaced solar plexus/abdominal aorta is one of
   the causes for constipation.
10. Take restful sleep for at least 6 hours daily.

Fasting once a week helps because the internal organs get rest from digestive functions and can focus on healing and correction processes.

Once we know the symptoms and understand the root causes, it is very easy to get rid of constipation for good with internal as well as external treatment methods suggested above. Introduce these changes step by step so they become habit over time. Start with what you can easily follow and experience relief and reversal of all discomfort.

3. HIGH BLOOD PRESSURE/HYPERTENSION

High B.P is a condition in which the force of the blood against the artery walls is high. Usually hypertension is defined as blood pressure above 140/90 and is considered severe if the pressure is above 180/120.

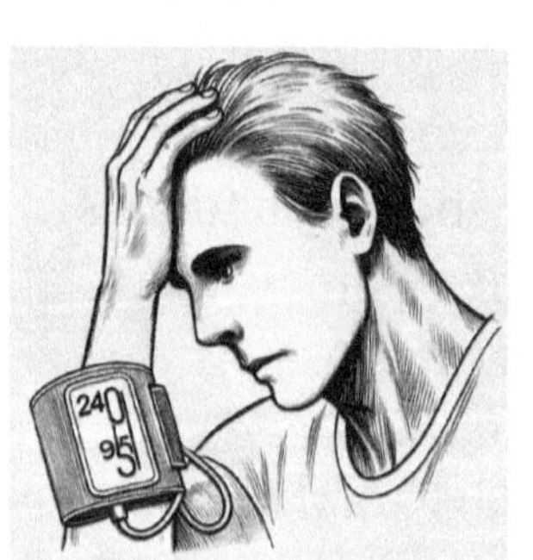

Symptoms
a) Reeling sensation in the head.
b) Pain in the backside of the head.
c) Constant headache.
d) Redness of eyes.
e) Continuous tension.

f) Increase in heart beat.
g) Sleeplessness.
h) Stroke in heart, brain.
i) Feeling of helplessness and lack of interest in anything.

Causes:

1. Stress is the main cause of hypertension.
2. Excess sugar and salt consumption through incorrect food choices.
3. Hardening of arteries and veins because of poor quality fats and oils in food.
4. Eating excessive animal based food.
5. Sedentary lifestyle.
6. Prolonged constipation.
7. Increase in blood urea levels
8. High acidic food consumption.
9. Diabetes.
10. Kidney malfunction.

Holistic treatment to rid hypertension involves internal and external measures.

Internal procedures

1. Alleviating stress with correct food, body and, mind practices.
2. Eating fiber rich carbohydrates like millets.
3. Drinking decoctions, early morning on empty stomach, made of leaves of basil, coriander and

giloy/amrita. Each type must be taken for a week.

4. Consuming juices made of ash gourd, bottle gourd, and cucumber. One type, weekly. The juice can be taken 30 minutes after the decoction.
5. Adding garlic in diet in the form of chutney or curries.
6. Cinnamon (*dalchini*) powder helps in reducing high BP.
7. Eating more alkaline food and reducing acidic food.
8. Drinking minimum of eight glasses of water daily.

External procedures

1. *Anulom Vilom* pranayama regularly for 15 minutes in a well-ventilated area brings down BP to normal range.

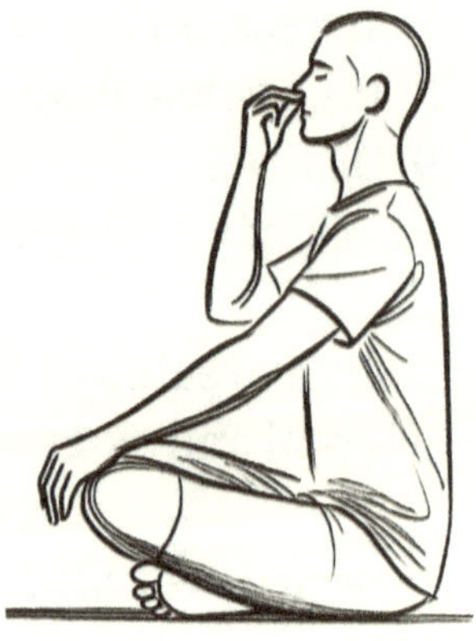

2. Other *pranayamas like chandra bhedhi, sheetali* and *sheetkari* help cool down the system.
3. Meditation for 15 minutes daily, morning and evening is helpful to center the mind and reduce stress.

4. *Yoga nidra* for 30 minutes helps give restful sleep thereby reducing high BP.

5. Walking for an hour in the morning in an oxygen-rich area supports circulation of blood in the entire body and has a cleansing effect.

6. Spinal bath for 5 minutes cools down the system instantaneously.

7. Cleaning the intestines through enema is akin to cleaning the silencer of a vehicle. Removal of toxins from the body with this powerful cleansing technique has a significant impact on reducing high BP.

Early and fast relief from high BP is necessary to prevent heart attack and brain stroke. The remedy is simple once we understand what our body needs to work well. We cannot be perfect 100% of the time but *we* know our body best. The next chapter elaborates on recognizing signs of illness. By staying tuned in to our body and identifying symptoms as they rise, we can catch a problem early. Complete reversal is initiated by making dietary changes because depending on what we choose, food and lifestyle are the biggest contributors to both disease and path to wellness. If food is right, no medicine is needed but no medicine is of use, if food is not right.

4. ASTHMA

Asthma is a condition in which a person's airways become inflamed, narrow, and produce extra mucus, making it difficult to breathe.

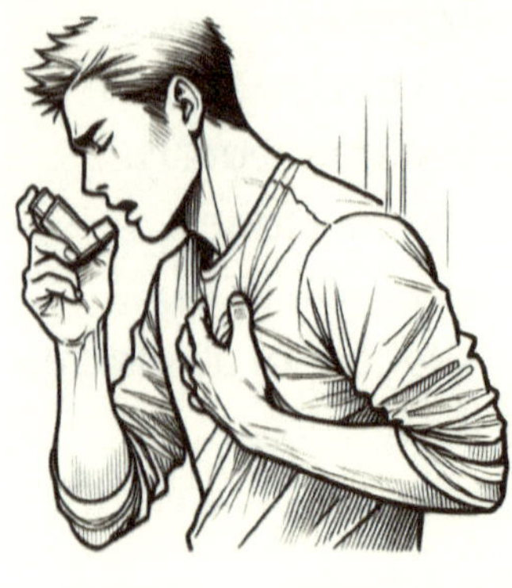

Ashtma can be minor or it can interfere with daily activities. In some cases, it may lead to a life-threatening attack.

Symptoms
1. Breathlessness.
2. Whistling breath.
3. Difficulty in breathing while lying down.
4. Worsened breathing in winter season.
5. Constant cough, sweating and redness in the face while coughing.
6. Cold hands and feet.

Causes
1. Eating fast foods, cold drinks, ice-cream, and refrigerated water.
2. Milk and milk products that are industrially processed and made mostly from genetically modified cows.
3. Refined cooking oils that are denatured by incorrect extraction methods aggravate *kapha*

and create imbalance in earth and water elements thereby blocking the respiratory system.
4. Consumption of sugar and refined flour/*maida* alter gut flora and the connection of the gut to all body systems significantly impacts performance of lungs.
5. Indigestion and constipation.
6. Spending long periods in air-conditioned environment.
7. Eating mostly acidic food.
8. Sedentary lifestyle and less oxygen intake.
9. Eosinophilia - increase in white blood cells in the blood.

Internal treatment

1. Reducing *kapha* in the body with the following food-based home remedies: a. Drinking *amla* or ginger juice in the morning. b. Consumption of raw garlic or garlic in curries or chutney. Allicin, a sulphur-containing compound in garlic gets rid of undesirable gut flora and also helps in reducing *kapha*. c. Licking one spoon of dry ginger powder with honey at night before sleep.
2. Consuming more natural and raw foods and less cooked food.
3. Wearing warm clothes and protecting the body from exposure to cold.

External treatment

1. Walking in sunlight for one hour or taking a sun bath.
2. Regular steam bath.
3. Inhalation of steam with turmeric powder.
4. Gargling with hot water with a little salt.
5. Enema gives relief by cleaning the bowels, preventing constipation and build-up of pathogenic gut flora.

6. Yoga asanas specific to Asthma- *bhujang, salabh, uttanasana, dhanur, paschimottasana, setubandh, ardh matsyendrasana, poorvauttanasana* and more.

7. *Surya bhedi, bhastrika,* and *nadi sodhan* pranayama help increase digestive fire in the body to melt away excess mucus and cleanse and balance the nervous system; *brahmri* pranayama helps increase nitric oxide that dilates airways.

8. *Jala neti* and *sutra neti* clean nasal passages and allow greater intake of oxygen.

The main goal of asthma treatment is to revive the respiratory system with natural remedies and preserve lung functioning. Asthma must be addressed in the initial stage itself. The pathways mentioned are clear and easy to follow and bring effective relief. Unlike medication, these methods strive to bring back the lost balance by getting rid of root cause.

5. DIABETES

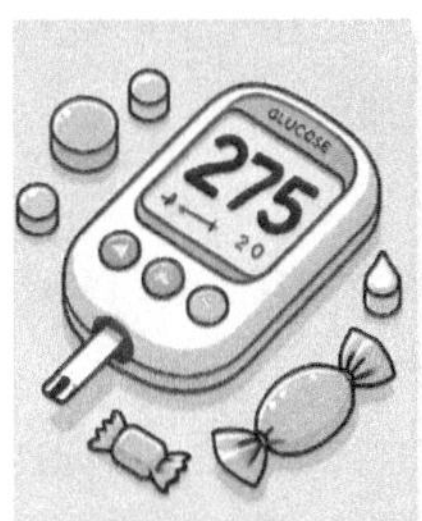

Diabetes is a chronic health condition where an imbalance is created in the cells because of excessive glucose in the body.

Food metabolism involves its breakdown into sugar (glucose) to get energy which is an essential need for the body. When glucose is released in the body, the pancreas immediately sends out insulin to remove it from the blood and pack it in cells where it can be broken down to release energy when needed. In this process water and carbon dioxide are also produced and eliminated by the body via kidneys and lungs. The other metabolic wastes are expelled via the bowels.

Insulin thus acts like a key - opening the door of cells so glucose can be sent in and stored for use. The problem rises when there is too much glucose entering the blood along with excess fat.

The body can safely handle upto 5-6 grams of glucose at a time in the blood but with far greater amounts entering in the form of simple carbohydrates, the pancreas has to continuously release insulin to clear away excess glucose. When this happens over an extended period, with too much insulin around all the time, the cells become insulin-insensitive and stop responding to its request to open doors. The amount of sugar tested in the blood begins to rise and the body enters the stage of pre-diabetes. If left unchecked, the sugar levels in blood rise even further indicating insulin insensitivity and high stress on the pancreas. This is called diabetes.

It is important to note here that insulin also regulates fat metabolism. It removes triglycerides and glucose from blood to be converted into fat in the liver, muscles and other tissues. The insulin is thus acting like a key for our muscle and liver cells too where fat gets stored. This is the fast way to reduce blood sugar. But if there is excess fat consumed or already present in the body this conversion process is impeded and levels of sugar lingering in the blood start rising. With animal fat there is more mayhem for the body but intake of plant based fat has to be balanced and controlled as well in order to brake and reverse diabetes.

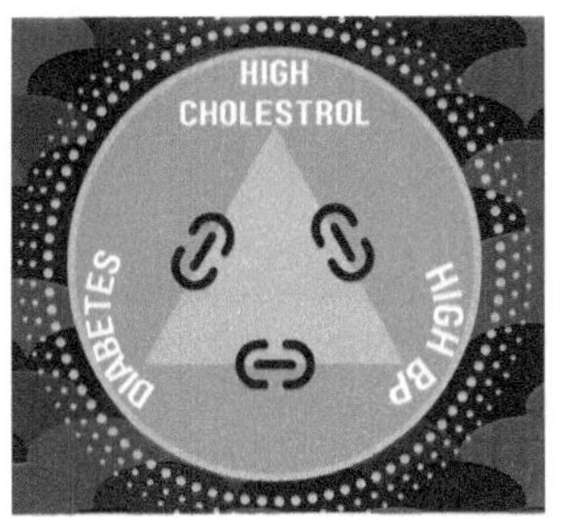

That is why diabetes is characterized by concomitant conditions of insulin insensitivity, high cholesterol and high blood pressure. High blood pressure is a result of narrowing of arteries with the fat and plaque deposits. Left uncorrected, the triangular trap of high sugar, cholesterol and blood pressure can lead to serious health problems involving vision, kidney and infection.

It is clear that the root cause here is continued release of glucose and fat in the blood which is worsened with high intake of fats. The culprits in diabetes clearly are low or no fiber foods like white rice, white flour/maida, sugar, products made of these, unrestrained intake of poor quality fats. Sedentary lifestyle, acidic foods, constipation and stress also contribute. Lastly, heredity can be a component but this switch can be kept 'off' by correct lifestyle and eating habits.

It is thus very important to amend eating habits and lifestyle choices at the earliest to reverse the condition. *Taking medicines to bring down blood sugar levels does not remove the sugar from the body. It only hides it in other places and precipitates damage there.*

Symptoms of pre-diabetes and diabetes

- Extreme tiredness.
- Sudden weight loss.
- Weakening eye sight.
- Heart weakness.
- Kidney problems.
- Nerves problems.
- Skin allergies.
- Pain in calf muscles.

Internal treatment

- Choose fiber rich grains, preferably small millets for lunch and dinner and avoiding paddy rice, wheat and foods containing them.
- Taking decoctions of leaves that support the pancreas and help control sugar metabolism. These are fenugreek, mint, coriander and, drumstick. Take one type every week and repeat the cycle. The decoctions must be taken early morning on empty stomach.
- Bitter gourd, *amla* and *methi* (fenugreek) juice.
- Jamun (Indian black berry) fruit.
- Take only natural food like sprouts, fruits, salads for breakfast.

External treatment
- Walking one hour daily in sunlight.
- Yoga asanas like *Mandukasana, Vakrasana, Gomukhasana, Bhastrika* pranayama, *Kapalbhati, Anulom Vilom* pranayama.
- Applying hot and cold packs alternately on the lower abdomen area activates pancreas.
- Spinal bath activates the nervous system and thereby the signaling process
- Tub bath activates intestines and helps remove constipation, if any.
- Dry massaging the body helps create heat in the body, stimulates blood circulation and digestion.

It is essential to reverse diabetes at the earliest in order to save the body from serious complications. High fiber carbohydrates, regular physical activity, decoctions of relevant leaves, getting proper sleep and managing stress are important factors which help reverse diabetes.

6. SINUSITIS

When the tissues lining the sinuses swell or become inflamed, it is called sinusitis. It occurs as a result of an inflammatory reaction or an infection from a virus, bacteria or fungus. It can also be a result of high intake of processed foods, dairy and animal protein that throws the immune system into disarray and creates allergic - hyper-immune- responses.

Symptoms

- Green or yellow discharge from the nose.
- Blocked nose.
- Pain and tenderness around cheeks, eyes or forehead.
- Reduced sense of smell.
- High temperature (fever).
- Ear pressure.
- Headache.
- Bad breath.

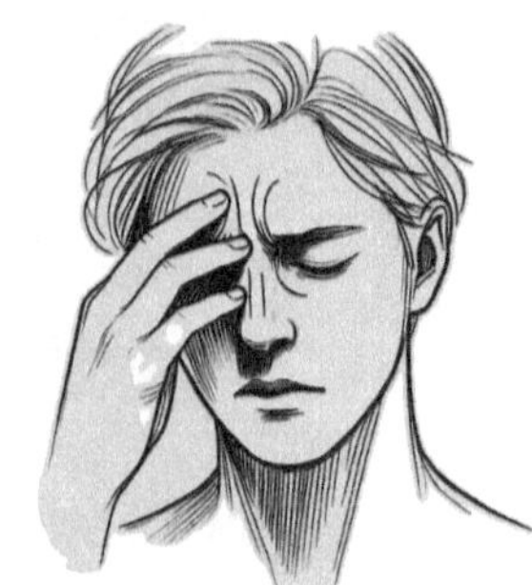

Cause

- Sinusitis is most often caused by common cold.
- Bacterial or viral infection.
- Smoking, or being around others who smoke.
- Low or altered immune response as a result of poor eating choices involving high intake of fried and processed foods, meat, sugar, and dairy.
- Deviated nasal septum. (Unless it is seriously off, there is a higher chance that above factors are implicated)

Internal Treatment

- Improving Vitamin C levels with mixed juice of *amla*, ginger and honey on empty stomach.

- Increasing *agni* or heat in the body through exercise and appropriate foods. Proper *agni* ensures proper digestion and reduces this *kapha* condition.
- Avoid all processed and mucus producing foods - milk and milk related products, paneer, ice cream, white flour/*maida*, sugar, cold water, cold drinks, animal based protein, sweets.
- Drink warm water only.
- Practice *Jala neti* and *Sutra neti*.
- Correct increased acidity in the body with dietary changes and natural therapies.

External Treatment

- Warm water bath only. Avoid cold water bath and head bath with cold water.
- Avoid air-conditioned environment which dries and irritates the sinus.
- Don't sleep directly under fan.
- Inhale steam by mixing turmeric powder in hot water.
- Wear warm clothes while going out and also cover head with a cap.
- Yoga practices that help - *Tadasana, Konasana, yoga mudra, bhujangasana, surya namaskar, anulom vilom pranayam.*

Sinusitis affects all age groups. It can accompany a wide range of conditions such as cough, asthma, headache and sore throat. Using medicines gives temporary relief only. Preventing recurrence and getting rid of it permanently involves getting rid of the root cause with natural treatment.

7. ACIDITY

Acidity is an imbalance often referred to as acid reflux or heartburn. It is a common digestive condition where stomach acid flows back into the esophagus, causing discomfort and a burning sensation in the chest. This condition is not always associated with over-production of stomach acid as is frequently thought. It can result from various factors, including dietary choices, lifestyle habits, and underlying medical issues. Understanding the triggers and management strategies for acidity is essential for maintaining digestive health and preventing long-term complications.

Symptoms
- Burning sensation in the stomach and throat.
- Burning sensation while passing urine.

- Severe pain in the lower chest area.
- Acid reflux.
- Gastritis.
- Peptic Ulcers.
- Indigestion.
- Constipation.
- Regurgitation.
- Excessive vomiting..
- Sleeplessness and restlessness.

Causes

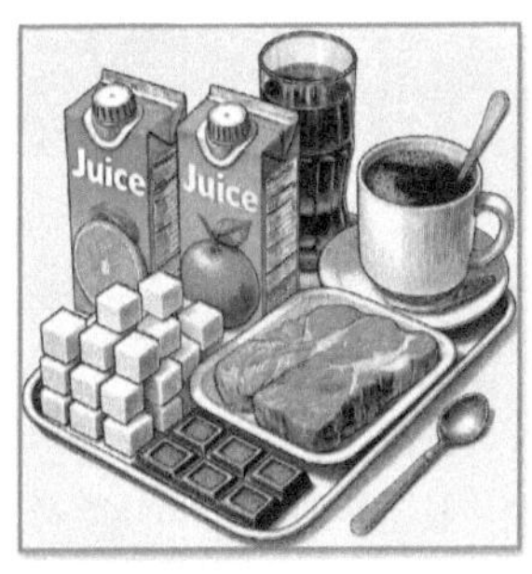

•*Dietary Habits*: Consuming a diet high in acidic and processed foods, sugars, and unhealthy fats can contribute to acidity. Trigger foods of acidity include eating *too much* of the following: animal protein and fatty cuts of meat; spicy foods like chili, hot sauce, peppers; citrus fruits and juices especially the processed varieties; carbonated and caffeinated beverages including coffee, tea, and some sodas; fried and fatty foods; tomato and ketchup; chocolate; alcohol particularly red wine, beer, and spirits.

- *Low Stomach Acid*: Stomach acid is crucial for the digestion of food, especially proteins, and for the absorption of nutrients. Contrary to the common belief that acidity is caused by too much stomach acid, low acid levels can lead to poor digestion and fermentation of food, which produces gas and pressure, causing acid to reflux into the esophagus. A sign of poor breakdown of food is undigested food in bowel like okra seeds, pieces of carrot or beet.

- **Stress** : Chronic stress, anger, fear and, negative emotions can negatively impact digestive function by altering the production of stomach acid and digestive enzymes. Stress can also lead to poor dietary choices and eating habits, exacerbating acidity.

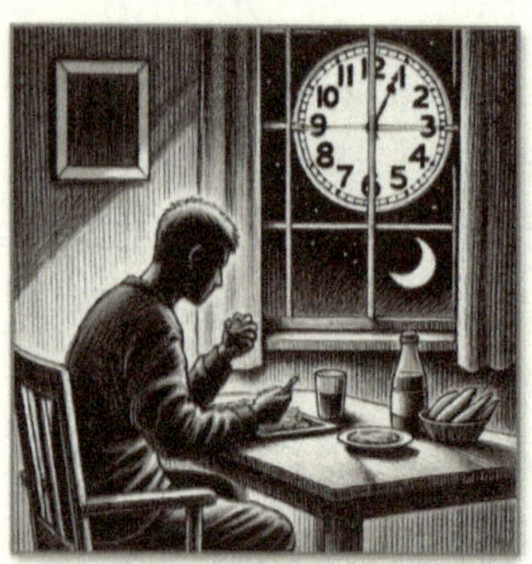

- **Poor Eating Habits**: Eating large meals, not chewing well, eating too quickly, or eating late at night can put pressure on the digestive system and lead to acid reflux.

- **Imbalance of Gut Flora**: Poor gut microbiome, like infection with H.pylori can affect digestion and contribute to symptoms of acidity. The kind of gut flora we have is in turn influenced by diet, antibiotic use, and overall health.

- **Food sensitivities**: Undiagnosed food sensitivities or intolerances (such as gluten or lactose intolerance) can lead to inflammation and digestive discomfort, including symptoms of acidity. Food sensitivity can happen due to pesticide and synthetic fertilizer use in growing food or due to poor gut flora.

- *Dehydration*: Insufficient water intake can lead to poor digestion and an increased risk of acidity.
- *Sedentary Lifestyle* : Lack of physical activity can slow down digestion and contribute to weight gain, both of which can increase the likelihood of experiencing acid reflux.
- *Structural Issues*: Conditions like hiatal hernia, where part of the stomach pushes through the diaphragm, can contribute to acid reflux and heartburn.

Treatment

Addressing the root cause of acid-related symptoms is key to treatment. Avoiding personal triggers and making dietary changes, lifestyle modifications are the natural remedies that reverse the condition without causing further distress.

Internal Work

1. Choose uncooked food like fruits, salads, and sprouts for breakfast.
2. Opt for smaller, more frequent meals.
3. Identify and avoid personal trigger foods.
4. Drink plenty of coconut water in the day.

5. Stay well hydrated with at least 8 glasses of
   water in the day.
6. One cup of cucumber, ash gourd, or bottle
   gourd juice on empty stomach in the morning.
7. Eat 80% alkaline food and less spicy food.
8. Eat food attentively, chewing well before
   swallowing.

External Treatment
- Apply mud pack or cold water cloth
  pack on the abdomen in the
  morning for 15 minutes.
- Tub bath for 15 minutes.
- Spinal bath.
- Enema to eliminate
  stools and clean colon
  regularly
- Yoga practices- *Sukshma vyayama,
  Chandrabhedi Seethali* and *Shitkari pranayama.*
- Reducing stress with meditation, walking, doing
  things one enjoys.
- Restful sleep for 6 to 8 hours.
- Yogic practices to fix hernia if that is the cause
  for acidity.

Acidity is a common condition that can cause
discomfort and pain. With lifestyle changes, one
can get relief, even reverse this malady. Taking
antacids might temporarily relieve symptoms but

it does not fix the problem and can be counterproductive in many situations. Where low acid is the cause, taking antacids impairs digestion and nutrient absorption even further. Some antacids, particularly proton pump inhibitors (PPIs), can cause a rebound effect where, after stopping the medication, the stomach produces even more acid than before. If poor gut flora is the cause, antacids mask the issue. Regular use of antacids can disrupt the body's natural acid-base balance, potentially leading to alkalosis, a condition where the body fluids have excess base (alkali) which can be even more dangerous.

8. THYROID

Thyroid conditions involve malfunction of the thyroid with imbalance in the amount of hormones secreted by the gland. Thyroid conditions can affect all age groups.

The main job of thyroid gland is to control the speed of metabolism. This is the process of transforming food into energy. All the cells in the body need energy to function. With metabolism impaired, thyroid patients feel constant weakness in the body.

The two main types of thyroid disease are hypothyrodism (under-active thyroid) and hyperthyroidism (over-active thyroid).

Symptoms
- Feeling tired (fatigue).
- Unexplained weight gain.
- Depressed mood.
- Sleeplessness.
- Sensitivity to heat.
- Feeling anxious, irritable or nervous.

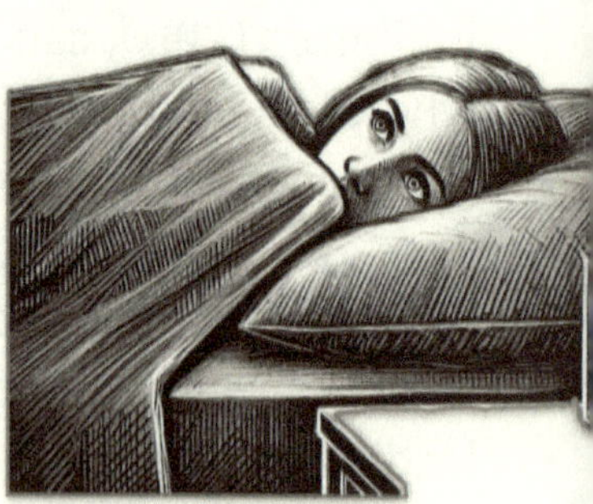

Causes
- Sedentary lifestyle.
- Viral infections.
- Stress.
- Poor dietary choices- eating fast/junk or toxic food.
- Sleep deprivation.
- Imbalance in gut health.
- Excessive sugar intake.

Internal Treatment
- Decoction of leaves - betel, *giloy*, drumstick - each one week on empty stomach in the morning.
- Consuming 3 teaspoon of oils - coconut, groundnut and, sesame- each type for 7 days and repeating the cycle. A gap of 30 minutes

must be there between decoction and oil. Glands need oils to function well therefore it is important to avoid refined oils and use only bull driven wooden *ghani* oil or cold pressed oil for cooking.

- Choosing fruits, salads and sprouts for breakfast and avoiding cooked food.
- Eating millet based food for lunch and dinner
- Chewing food well for proper digestion and supporting metabolism.

External Treatment

1. All neck exercises because the movement massages the thyroid and infuses fresh blood into it. Beneficial yoga asanas for the thyroid are- *bhujangasan, sarvangasan, halasan, ushtrasan, mandukasan, markatasan* and, *pawan muktasana.*

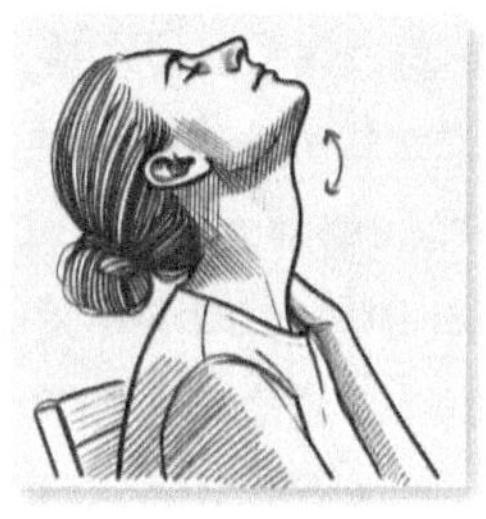

2. *Pranayama - Ujjayi pranayam* 21 times both morning and evening. *Simhasan* (Lion roaring) 1 to 2 minutes.

3. Accupressure - Pressing thyroid point (just below the thumb) for two minutes on each hand, morning and evening.

The above mentioned treatment works for both hypo and hyperthyroidism. Thyroid conditions are reversed by restoring the imbalance through natural treatment. Holistic therapies corrects all aspects that impact thyroid function - food, movement, lifestyle- and removes all blockages to energy flow to cure the problem with no side effects. It is possible to correct thyroid disease even after years of medication provided the treatment is followed properly and the medicines phased off gradually under guidance of a supportive doctor.

9. SKIN PROBLEMS

Skin is the largest organ in the human body. It is a protective shield that takes the brunt from outside and safeguards other organs. Although most skin diseases manifest in the layers of the skin, diagnostic assessments reveal connections to internal health issues. The condition of the skin signals possible internal imbalances. Observing and recognizing changes in the skin helps in detecting internal problems sooner and in treating both the surface issue and root cause.

In this chapter simple, proactive home remedies are suggested for common skin problems that are effective and easy to follow.

Symptoms

- Rashes with itchiness or pain.
- Dry skin
- Peeling skin
- Scaly or rough skin
- Red, white or pus-filled bumps

Causes

- Contact with allergens
- Dominance of pathogenic gut flora- fungus, parasites and, bacteria
- Low or altered immunity
- Exposure to extreme climatic conditions.
- Unhygienic practices and condition of the body
- Stress

Internal Treatment

- Decoctions of aloe vera, mint, chamomile, and, coriander leaves - One week each type taken empty stomach in the morning. Repeat the cycle till the condition clears.
- Stopping all acidic and animal based food.
- Avoid salty food and all sour fruits.
- Eating natural food with emphasis on fresh produce and whole grains.
- Detox the body with Ayurveda, Siddha or Nature Cure therapy.

- Ensure growth and dominance of beneficial gut flora with right fermented foods daily like small millets *ambali* and goat milk kefir.

External Treatment
- Daily sesame oil application to the affected area.
- Herbs like *Wrightia tinctoria, Indigofera tinctoria and Indigofera aspalathoide* infused in coconut oil and applied on the affected skin have been found to be helpful in psoriasis by reducing inflammatory reactions by keeping the skin moisturized and maintaining the water-oil balance in cells.
- Applying neem/basil leaves paste on rashes.
- Mud bath or mud pack application.
- Allowing sufficient air circulation to the skin by wear cotton clothes.
- Avoid using toiletries with chemicals on the skin. Choose soaps, creams, lotions, fragrant sprays that are completely free of chemicals that interfere with cell and endocrine gland function.
- Reduce stress by following correct lifestyle practices.

Home remedies suggested here are for mild skin diseases accompanied by itchiness, dry skin or rashes. It is important to adopt proper skin hygiene, lifestyle changes and consult a skilled ayurvedic or naturopathic practitioner in aggravated conditions.

10. URINE PROBLEMS

Urinary problems are usually expressed as need to urinate frequently or in urine burning sensation. Many people, especially the elderly suffer from this problem. Bed wetting is common in children. Let us understand the causes within the framework of holistic approach.

In Ayurveda *Vata* dosha governs movement and flow in the body. An imbalance in *Vata* can lead to issues like frequent urination, urinary retention, and pain during urination. Causes might include dehydration, excessive stress, and a diet high in dry or cold foods. *Pitta* dosha is associated with heat and metabolism. An imbalance in Pitta can lead to burning sensations during urination, inflammation, and infections such as urinary tract infections (UTIs). This is often caused by excessive intake of spicy, sour, or acidic foods, dehydration, and emotional stress. *Kapha* dosha relates to structure and lubrication in the body. An imbalance in *Kapha* can cause sluggish urinary function, leading to issues like retention and formation of kidney stones. Causes include a sedentary lifestyle, excessive intake of sweet or oily foods, and lack of exercise all of which lead to stagnation of blood in the lower abdomen which can obstruct the urinary passages, leading to painful and difficult urination. The fourth important force that is always checked in Ayurveda is digestive fire or *agni*. Weak digestive fire can lead to the accumulation of toxins (*Ama*) in the body, which can obstruct urinary channels and lead to problems.

Since kidneys play a crucial role in water metabolism and control the opening and closing of the bladder it is logical that deficiency in kidney energy will lead to all urinary problems. Simple remedies exist that can be used successfully to restore balance and energy.

Frequent Urination

- Consume sweet *laddu* made of 50gm black sesame, 25gm *ajwain*/carom seeds and 50gm jaggery - morning and evening daily. For children, reduce it to half.
- Eat two bananas daily because it is a good source of minerals needed for kidney and bladder function. The fiber in it supports bowel movement and prevents constipation which can put pressure on bladder and increase frequency of urination.

- Have 100gm grapes morning and evening for one week.
- Apply hot pack/pad below the navel for 10 minutes in the evening.
- Avoid drinking excessive water, especially close to bedtime.

Burning sensation during urination

- Have cucumber juice - 1 cup in the morning on empty stomach.
- Bottle gourd juice with honey- 1 cup in the morning on empty stomach.
- Soak one tsp coriander seeds in water overnight and drink the water next morning. The left-over seeds can be used for composting.
- Apply cold pack on abdomen for 15 minutes in the evening.
- Take cold water immersion (tub bath) for 15 minutes
- Avoid spicy food.

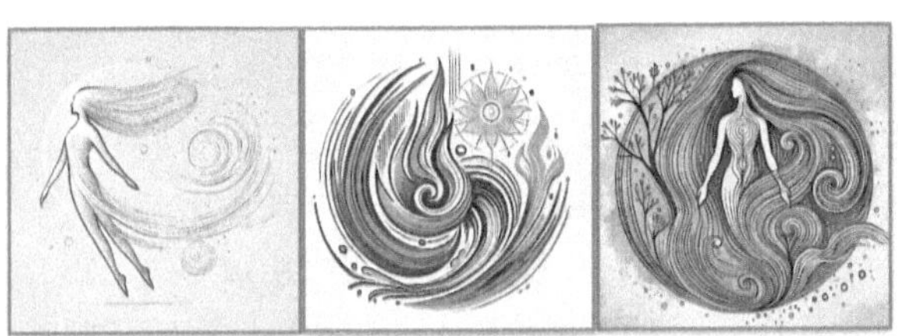

16

Signs & Signals

The body is naturally designed to move towards balance. In its progression towards equilibrium it gives distress signals that can be picked easily if we are attuned to the signs. The aim of this chapter is to familiarize ourselves with some of these cues. They might look simple but picking them up early than later can save us lot of trouble. Prolonged neglect can result in serious consequences to health so it is best we learn to read our body well.

No disease or illness develops overnight. Most diseases are caused by breaching the laws of nature - ignoring her rules, indulging in wrong eating and drinking habits, poor choices like smoking and alcohol, over-burdening organs and neglecting fundamental rules of hygiene. These can lead to disturbances in the body that are indicated in some of the following ways.

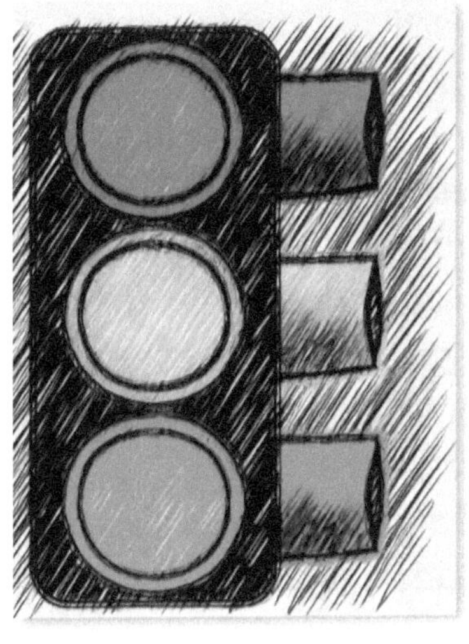

1. ***Urine and bowel movement*** are strong indicators of disharmony. Less urination and insufficient bowel movement causes toxins to accumulate in the body. Increased urination on the other can be a sign of increased levels of sugar in the blood.

2. Reduced ***appetite*** and improper ***digestion*** of food which can be detected in undigested particles of food in stool (pieces of carrot or seeds of okra/lady-finger). It may be accompanied by constipation or loose motions. All these are signs of reduced digestive fire in the stomach, congestion in the body and under performing digestive system.

3. ***Skin*** issues which is a result of impurity of blood. There can be other reasons but it is often a natural consequence of the two reasons listed above. This also illustrates the connectedness of our body- how one thing leads to another and the role of proper diagnosis based on this inter-connection. While the symptom might be skin issue the cause can

be malfunctioning digestive system and a linked kidney problem.

4. ***Mouth breathing*** because of which blood is not oxygenated properly and carbon dioxide is not cleared from the organs. The result is accumulation of toxins that can lead to many problems including high blood pressure. It must be noted and corrected in everyone including babies and children.

5. ***Fatigue*** and reduced vitality is also a sign of increased carbon dioxide and toxins that leads to slow functioning of organs and further buildup of waste in the body.

6. ***Frequent illness*** or vulnerability to germs or disease is a sign of weakened immune function. This is a result of poor habits, growth of fake foods and industrial agriculture that is affecting our immunity and gradually performance of all systems.

7. ***Prolonged or chronic illness*** can be a sign of disturbed endocrine system. Usually the thyroid/parathyroid gland is the first endocrine gland thrown off balance and gradually all other glands are affected.

8. ***Ache or pain*** in any particular part indicates blocked energy flow or congestion of carbon dioxide, water and air.

9. ***Runny nose*** and sneezing mean the body is trying to throw out excess water.

10. **Coughing** indicates that the body is feeling cold and that it is trying to clear congestion in the throat and the chest.
11. **Itching** shows that a greater flow of blood is required around that part.
12. **Fever** indicates battle in our body between white blood cells and germs.
13. **Twisting** of the body indicates that it is tired and requires rest and oxygen.
14. Pain or murmur in the **heart** indicates that the heart requires total rest.

Before treating any condition, we should understand these signals of our body. It is counter-productive to stop them suddenly by using drugs. For example fever is usually a sign of the body fighting an infection. So unless the fever is very high, stopping it can result in development of another problem.

In order for our immune and endocrine system to work well, focus needs to be on improving their function with time-tested medicinal herbs, establishing organic farming practices and supporting the body to over-power pathogens rather than taking antibiotics and experimental drugs. The latter has resulted in mutation of pathogens into anti-biotic resistant and other ever-changing vicious forms.

Over-eating is a common habit that over-loads the system and drains energy. We can easily avoid this if we are attentive to the belching signals the body gives. As we ensure intake of proper nutrition on a daily basis, waste accumulation must be prevented with easy and economically accomplished periodic cleansing. We will be better off paying heed to simple, natural signals for thirst, hunger, urination, bowel movement, and develop a habit of looking beyond our image.

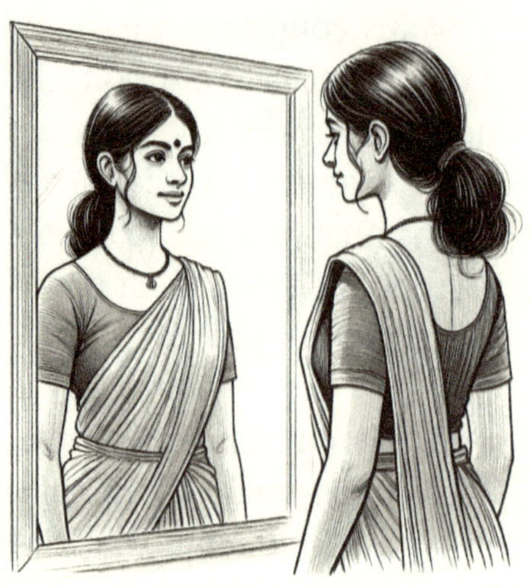

17

Tips

Good health is a direct result of three practices :

1. Clean the body periodically.
2. Stop intake of items that compromise balance.
3. Follow habits that rebuild and maintain wellness.

Although covered in earlier chapters it helps to glean out the key components and group them here for easy reminder. Let's take a look.

Clean accumulated toxins and waste matter. The method to accomplish this is simple. Increase intake of water (at least 8 glasses), raw food and juices on a daily basis. Mini, home-based *panchkarma* can be done with every change in season. Some of the practices include

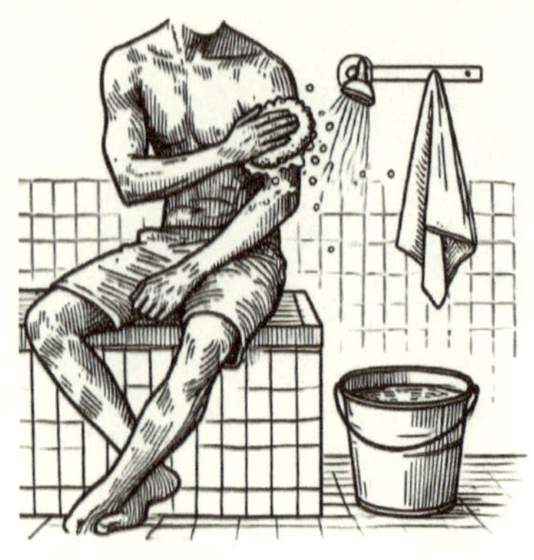

massaging with oil, cleaning the colon with enemas, and the upper digestive tract with *Kunjal Kriya* - drinking salt water and inducing vomiting. Enema can also be done once every week. If not, make sure it's done periodically. It is safe and with the amount of toxicity around us, very beneficial. Cleansing supports the body in detoxing and lifts the burden off the cells.

Stop everything that throws the body off balance.

Choose nourishing, nature made food. Factory produced food and drinks have ingredients whose safety is not tested and are in fact associated with serious health risks. They lower immunity and are at the root of growing allergies. Continued intake of these items masquerading as food, slowly builds toxicity in the body and leads to chronic and even serious conditions. They are therefore best avoided.

Refined oils should be emptied from our pantries since they are denatured, contain toxic chemicals and damage function of our cells.

Avoid microwave oven cooking, air-fryers, aluminum and non-stick pots and pans. Also consider that cooking on high heat kills the nutrients in food so prefer low heat and slow cooking.

Follow habits that rebuild and maintain wellness.

For cooking choose safe or natural materials to cook in like cast iron, steel, clay pots and utensils. Pick naturally extracted, bull-driven, wood pressed or second best, cold-pressed oils. Local oils like mustard, sesame, coconut, safflower and ground nut are preferred.

Maintain a schedule. Eat on time and while eating, chew food thoroughly in the mouth before swallowing so it can mix with digestive enzymes present in the saliva. The first step in digestion takes place in the mouth so ensuring a longer stay there is very helpful in food breakdown and nutrition absorption process.

Replace white sugar, factory salt, and white flour/ *maida* with jaggery, sea salt or pink salt, and whole grains like millets.

Sleep on time and take rest breaks through the day. Choose a lifestyle that allows the proverbial

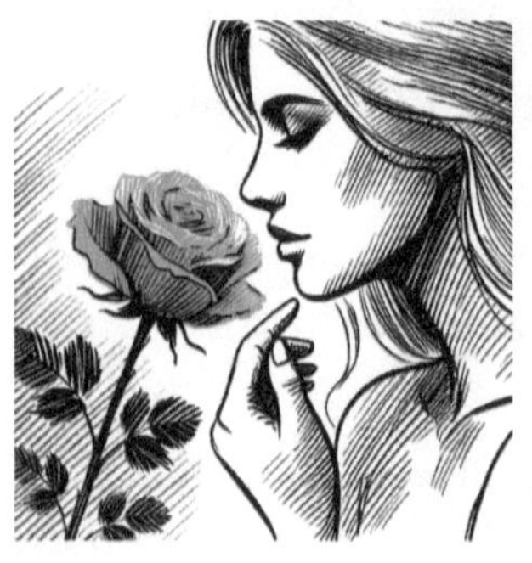

'smelling the roses'. Rest rejuvenates and charges the body and brain. At night avoid sleeping immediately after eating and build the habit of getting up early in the morning.

As already discussed, massaging the body with oil frequently and exposing the skin to sunshine for sometime before taking a bath maintains wellness. It moisturizes and nourishes the skin and also provides the body with essential vitamin D.

Being out in the Sun for at least half-an-hour every day ensures free supply and quota of Vitamin D. Sunshine obtained in morning and evening hours is safe and does not cause any sunburn or damage.

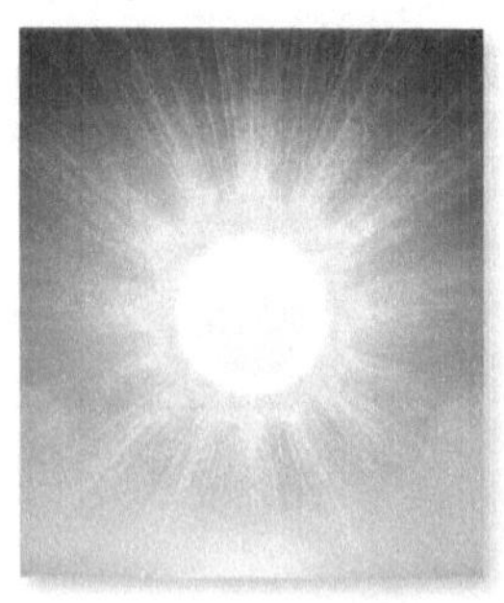

Never suppress the urge to urinate or defecate. This is a signal from the body to get rid of waste and must be followed immediately. Do some physical activity daily that makes the body sweat. Our skin is the largest cleansing organ and its pores are a way to release waste. Exercise induced sweat takes the load off the kidneys and easily gets rid of waste material

Acute conditions like fever, cold, cough, diarrhoea, dysentery, and skin eruptions should not be suppressed unless they pose a risk. They are a way to rid waste and help the body to recover. Elect to use simple remedies as outlined in chapter 3, to alleviate these symptoms aligned to nature's ways of healing and restoring health.

Develop the habit of deep breathing. There are energizing and balancing practices in breathing that if done regularly, channel the life force or *pran-shakti* to every cell in the body. Some of these are *bhastrika, anulom-vilom, kapalbhati, ujjayi, brahmri* and *udgeet. Pranayama* for 15-30 minutes everyday helps instant uptake of oxygen by the body.

Walking bare-feet on the soil daily is an easy detox for the body. It releases free radicals into the ground, healing the body at the cellular level.

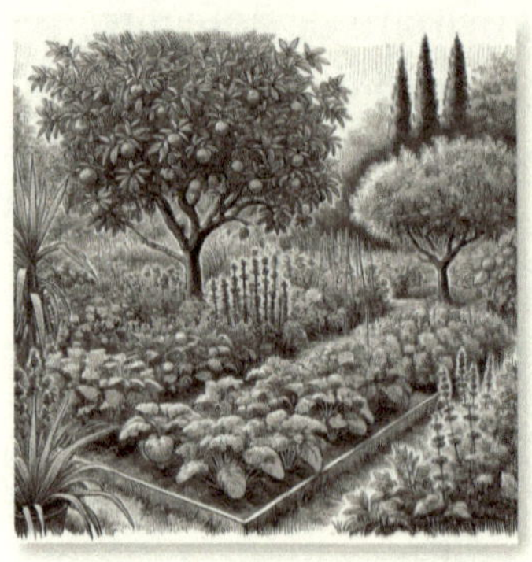

Maintain a kitchen garden and also grow medicinal herbs in it. Container gardening is possible in small spaces. A community garden can be built and maintained for all to enjoy. Tulsi, drumstick, papaya, mango, neem, guava, orange, lemon, curry leaves, herbs, vegetables and greens can be easily grown. Make sure the soil around the house and your community is kept microbe rich with natural fertilizers, wood mulch and compost made of your kitchen waste. Gardening nurtures the earth and also becomes a source of interaction, comfort and pleasure for everyone.

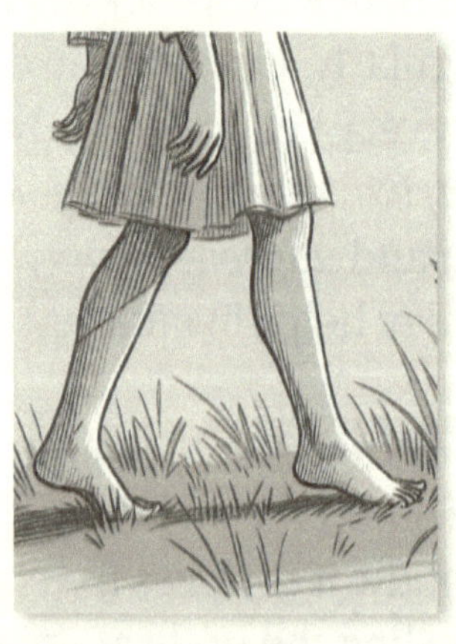

Part 2

1

Mind Power

When striving for a disease-free life, understanding the physical body is going half way through. Scientific wisdom evident in time-tested health practices of India mention clearly that the body itself is

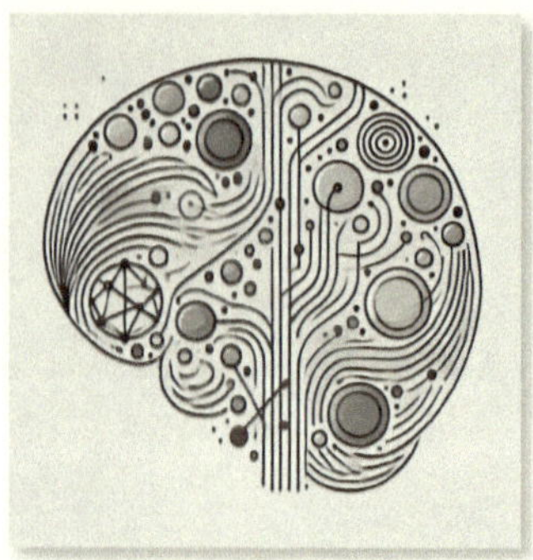

rooted or strongly linked to the mind that lies atop. Diseases germinate in the terrain of the mind as thought waves and get manifested in the physical body below. They thus have a psychosomatic

dimension. *Psyche* meaning mind and *soma* the physical body.

There is two way interaction between the mind and body. Both influence and exercise control over each other. A happy and healthy body can be maintained only in a happy and healthy mind and vice versa. Thus for good health we need to have both working simultaneously in the right way. So far we have learnt how to take care of the body (*Soma*). We will now attempt to know the mind (*Psyche*) and how it functions and exerts its influence.

Bulk of the problems we face are initiated and aggravated by stress. For sure our ability to handle stress is determined by the nourishment we put in the body and the presence of key nutrients needed by both the brain and body. However, stress absorption and processing is also dependent on our

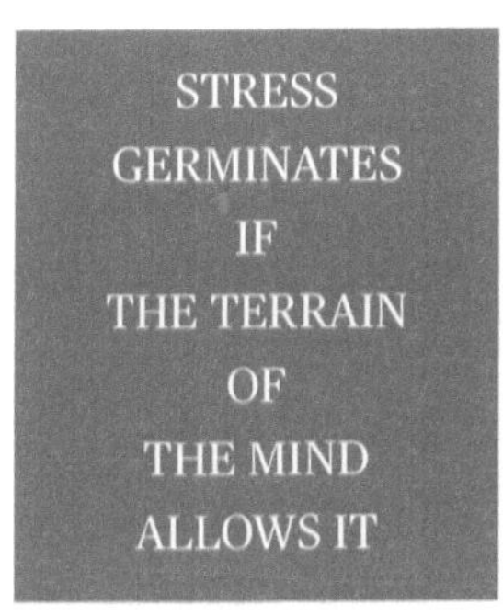

emotional complexion. Stress germinates if the terrain of the mind allows it. It is in fact, it's creation. The emotional colors or drivers that birth and drive stress are primarily worry and fear but anger, greed, and ego play significant roles as well.

Coming straight to the point, health and happiness of the mind can be achieved by abandoning all worries, fears and standing a strong guard over our negative emotions. If a list is made of them, we will be surprised most are unwarranted.

However, in the modern world, almost everyone is beset with worry, fear, and emotions that pull us down and so consequently we feel great mental stress. Unfortunately, stress affects directly and indirectly not only the person harboring it but has a ripple effect, affecting most of his/her immediate family members. Modern lifestyle itself is a cause of mental stress.

W.H. Auden, an english poet, said, "Twentieth Century is an age of anxiety." Looking around, we are ascertained of this. Everyone suffers from some level of anxiety or mental stress both within and outside the home. Our great-grand parents and grand-parents lived healthy and happily since they were saved from the levels of stress we witness today. The normal strain and pressures they faced were warded off with natural, nourishing foods and a life supported by adequate emotional network.

Today the structure of life is such that everyone-students, housewives, employees, business people, even young children - is racing on roller wheels, burdened with stress that slowly erodes health and lowers quality of life even as it purportedly extends it. From the time we wake up until bedtime, we suffer mental pressure, anxiety, and high blood pressure. How does this happen? Let us examine this a little deeply picking a sample life of an Indian housewife, mistakenly viewed as one lacking any strain or pressure. Some tweaks will be needed to adjust for local realities, but generally speaking, it can be considered to be globally relevant.

Stress of a Housewife

A day for a typical Indian housewife might start on a distressed note. Perhaps unable to sleep well due to mosquitos at night, she is upset early morning by the normal bell of the milkman and the noise in the street. She has to get the children ready for school.

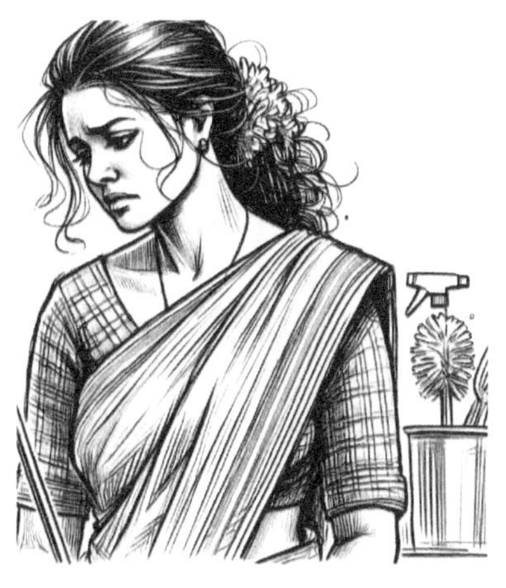

Everything needs to be ready for the husband to leave for office. When she tries to get some respite later, perhaps some neighbour, friend or relative drops in. The cell phone is constantly ringing and although most calls are unnecessary she feels the anxiety of missing an important call.

Meanwhile, the gas boy rings the bell. If she doesn't attend to him, she will miss the gas cylinder. A courier boy comes to deliver an article. Some people may disturb her by enquiring about the address of a person on the street. Somehow she finishes the cooking and work in the house. Now she is anxious about taking a bath peacefully lest someone knock on the door. The bath over, she could possibly squeeze in a nap to shrug off the tiredness but looking at the the clock she realizes it is time for the children to return from school. She has to take care of them. Later, the husband comes back. She has to handle demands by children for their choice of food and special attention requested by the husband. Everything over, it is 11 p.m. She wishes to sleep but the mosquitos start buzzing!

A Competitive World For All

The story of stress doesn't just engulf one section or population of society today. It has deluged everyone, including the very young ones. While in school children are stressed by examinations and their performance. After studies they face terrible anxiety about securing a job. When job is secured, the stress shifts to procuring things one by one on installments and EMIs. Then marriage happens, either by choice or selection by parents.

Then follows the seeming problem of adjusting with another person as a husband or wife. Not so easy, either love or arranged marriage! If they do not have children that is one problem but after having children, other problems follow!

Financial Stress

A perpetual source of frustration for the modern man is the constant lagging of income behind expenditure. There is a mountain load of loans, credit card payments, and EMIs overwhelming everyone. As the cost of everything rises continuously, so do our desires and wants.

Is it possible then to live a stress-free, peaceful life in these circumstances that are seemingly engulfing all from west to east?

The answer is a positive and strong yes.
There are several solutions for relief from stress.
Let us go through some in the following chapters.

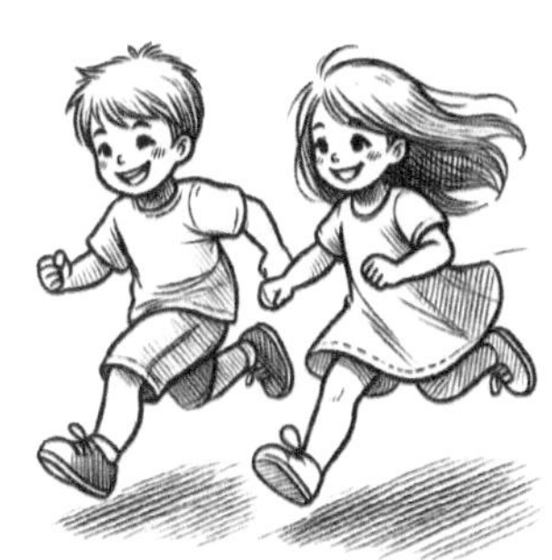

2

Reprogramming the Mind

Our mind is a computer that has been programmed at birth. We respond in the way we do because of this mental wiring. We are at the mercy of the way our mind has been conditioned (programmed) to act.

The root cause of all chronic tension lies in our emotional reaction to people and situations around us which is determined by this conditioning. The solution, therefore, is to change the program in our brain and rewire it so that we do not respond in a negative way when we face a trigger situation. Even though this cannot be achieved overnight, with a little patience and practice we can succeed.
So how do we re-program the mind? Some techniques that are helpful and work are as follows:

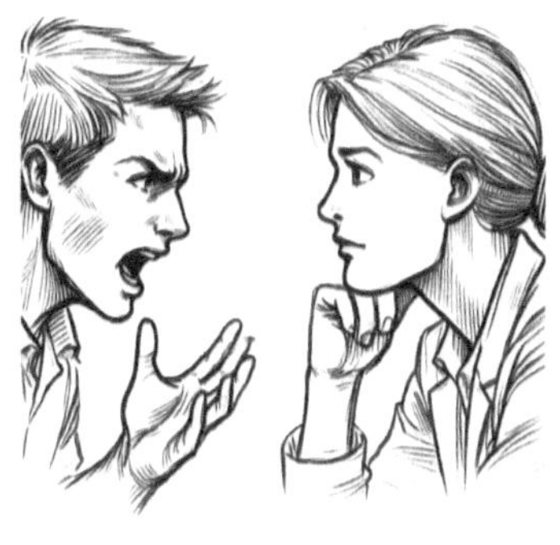

1. ***Accept other people*** fully knowing they have reasons to think and behave the way they do because of *their* own mental conditioning. Looking at this another way, if possible, try to put yourself in their shoes and we might get some insights to their reasons to act and say what they do. Trying to see the other person's point of view will in fact help us navigate an unpleasant situation better and have a high chance of leading to a favorable and acceptable outcome for all concerned.

2. ***Accept yourself*** along with your unique strengths and situation. They are not necessarily your limitations. It is our inability to accept ourselves and the matrix we are in that causes so much unnecessary anguish in life. If we dislike our situation and it can be improved there is reason for us to put in the work to do so in a pleasant way. If not, we are better off accepting gracefully and positively what we have and keep striving.

Nothing is permanent and things change sooner with a positive mindset than we think.

3. ***Accept what you fail to get*** with a sense of detachment rather than fret and fume. Logically speaking frustration does not achieve anything. It is time to put forward one foot after another and move on.

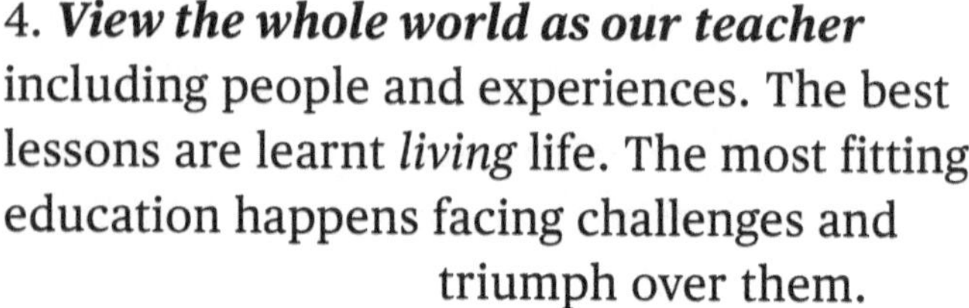

4. ***View the whole world as our teacher*** including people and experiences. The best lessons are learnt *living* life. The most fitting education happens facing challenges and triumph over them.

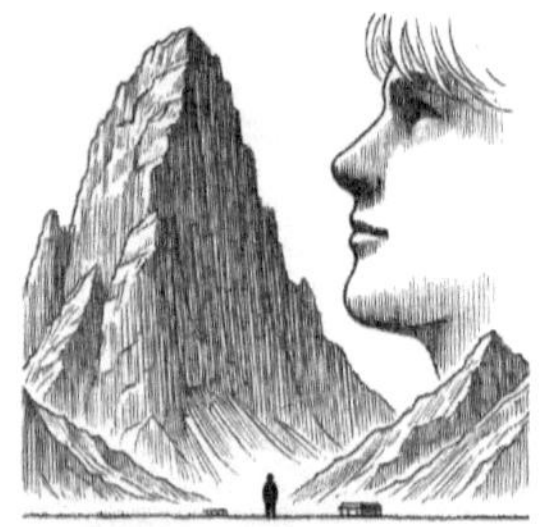

5. ***Live every moment and enjoy every action*** therein. See the profound in the mundane and joy in simple, repetitive acts of daily life. By fully engaging with the present we are often surprised with astonishing insights that sometimes change the course of our life.

6. ***We are consciousness (awareness) first***. When we believe that, we are not limited to our

body and mind and try to go beyond physical limitations. We live more and more in awareness of our 'conscious' reality we learn to use a force that remains neglected and unspoken.

7. ***Let us not be what we are not***. If we try to be what we are not, when trying to impress people, we immediately experience mental tension. The easy solution is : Don't attempt it. Just be your own self. Oscar Wilde funnily said, "Be yourself; everyone else is already taken." It is only when we act and speak what we are, we develop self-confidence and make genuine connections with others and as a result learn more about ourself and the world around.

8. ***Treat difficult situations as the greatest teachers*** and do not try to avoid them. Typically we run or hide from uncomfortable environments, but if we changed this approach and actually face them, we will be surprised how easily they defuse and resolve.

When we start reprogramming our mind with these strategies, gradually but surely, our attitude to others and ourselves starts shifting. We may not be able to rewire everything but it is possible to start with one and slowly, lets say every month add a new way of thinking. Every change will naturally thwart negative reactions which is the typical cocktail stress is made of. Refusing to fill our mind with this cocktail keeps the interior confines of the mind clean and clear. Stress is thus kept at bay and we feel healthy and happy. This is the fuel that keeps us going.

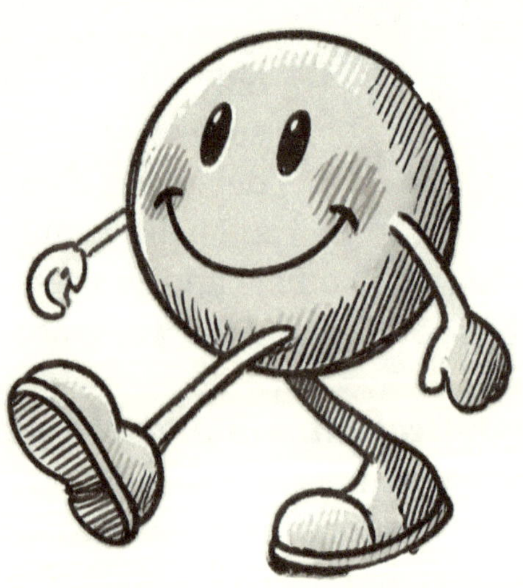

3

Body-Work for the Mind

Just as we can reprogram our thoughts and make new grooves in the terrain of the mind, we can ward off undesirable thought patterns or stress that originates in the mind with the help of the body. Yoga is excellent at relaxing both the mind and the body. *As the body relaxes, it signals the mind to relax*. Relaxation has a strong inverse relationship with stress.

Relaxation releases tension from both the mind and body to allow complete rest and revitalization. This is the ideally the task of sleep. However, because our life is rife with tension, sleep no longer performs its function properly. Sleep is still necessary, not replaceable, but it needs to be supplemented with powerful yoga techniques that quickly and efficiently remove worry and stress and lead the body to a state of total relaxation.

Yoga offers some much needed relaxation techniques through asanas, pranayama and meditation.

Asanas

It may seem surprising, but the first step in attaining deep relaxation through asanas is to tense the whole body. It is only after applying muscular tension to the entire body that we can subsequently allow our whole body to relax. Relaxing the body-mind complex also helps relieve and prevent diseases. Here are some asanas that if done properly and regularly, help us diminish strain and attain rest.

Naukasana

Naukasana or boat pose is a good asana for relaxing many muscles and joints of the body - the abdomen, lower back, and legs. It helps bring immediate relief to those people suffering from nervousness and tension. *Naukasana* takes between 3- 4 minutes.

Shavasana & Yog Nidra

Deadman's pose, *shavasana* relaxes the whole physiological-psychological system by releasing strain from the whole body, part by part and breathing vital energy or *prana* into them with focussed attention. *Yog Nidra* is another powerful technique similar to *Shavasana*. With the mind relaxed we are able to see and relate to the world and people around us in a more comfortable way, conduct our work more smoothly and experience more happiness. *Shavasana* and *Yog Nidra* can be done anytime you feel a need to lie down and rest.

Pranayama

Pranayama is expansion of *prana* or the vital force. A few minutes of yogic breathing daily can work wonders. Just as a bath cleanses the body, *pranayama* purifies blood and the mind, making us less susceptible to illness. We acquire more power, vitality and calmness in our daily activities. By inhaling the full amount of oxygen with these powerful breathing exercises we boost circulation of nutrients which helps in developing clarity in thinking.

There are different techniques of breathing each with its own set of benefits. As one transitions to making pranayama part of daily life, we can slowly add the range of techniques.

Bhastrika or bellows breath supplies the body with large amount of *prana vayu* (vital energy air) and gets rid of impure air (carbon dioxide) at the same time. When done correctly, *bhastrika* helps control the mind, increase concentration and vanquish laziness.

Anulom-Vilom purifies the nerves and therefore strengthens the nervous system. It is also very beneficial in ailments of the lungs and hypertension.

In *Kapalbhati* the focus is on forceful exhale and abdominal gases are thrown out with vigor. This increases power of concentration as impurities are removed from the nerves of the skull region.

Ujjayi pranayama removes ailments of the throat, nose and ear and hence cold and cough.

Brahmari or the buzzing bee pranayama generates vibrations that massage and strengthen tissues of the brain. It keeps the mind alert and with regular practice becomes a spiritual experience.

Regular and increasing time given to each pranayama brings commensurate gains to the mind, body and spirit.

Meditation

Meditation is another way to overcome mental disturbances and calm the mind and body. It is as simple as sitting in silence and watching one's breath or thoughts. With constant noise surrounding us today, this is an almost essential practice to tune into oneself. It can be done by anyone irrespective of age.

Although there is no instant success here, consistent practice leads to success in detaching all happiness from sense objects and in gaining some control over the mind. Meditation is not just for yogis and sadhus. Everyone, including children, is benefitted from it. An achievable goal is at least 10 minutes of meditation daily at dawn and dusk.

The requirements for meditation are few and easy. Just a clean space, comfortable posture, seat and regularity. There are several forms of meditation each with its own merit. One can be meditative doing asanas, focussing on the stretches and their effect on the body. Pranayama can be meditative with the mind watching the in and outflow of breath. Meditation can be observation or creation of one's thoughts as they flow in and out. One can create an idea, dwell over it for a few seconds, then let it go, to allow another idea to emerge.

Om chanting is another powerful form of meditation with focus centered on the center of the eyebrows.

Tratak of the sun is a great way to meditate. It is done by gazing at the orange rays of the sun shortly before sunrise and sunset. These are suffused with light frequencies that improve the body's Vitamin-D levels and positively affect several physiological processes including immunity. Besides being good for our eyes it calms the mind and uplifts the spirit. Take care to not look at the sun directly any other time.

All forms of meditation help. Those who suffer from insomnia, confidence or get agitated and worried easily will find stability and control over the mind which is the root cause of these problems.

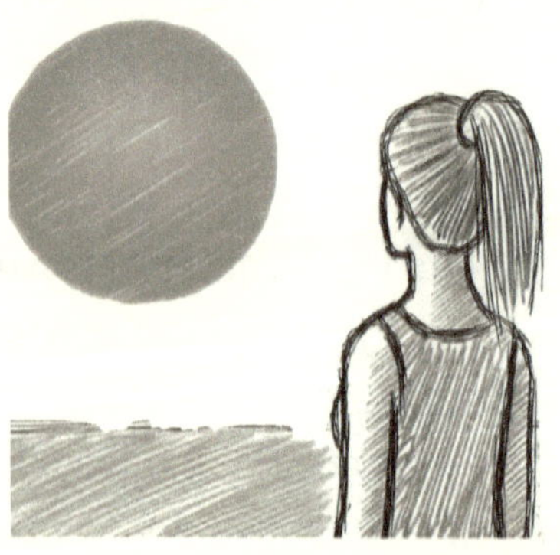

Inner peace, stress reduction, awareness, mental clarity, resilience, and emotional balance are natural outcomes of meditation. It's profound ability to transform both mind and body come to everyone that practices.

Practical training of Yoga Techniques

Initially yoga techniques should be learned from an experienced yoga teacher. A short, guided training for a month is sufficient to get started if the determination exists. Thereafter, one can easily practice at home. Of course, practicing in a group is motivating and can ensure continuity. Either way, the benefits are enormous and well worth the investment.

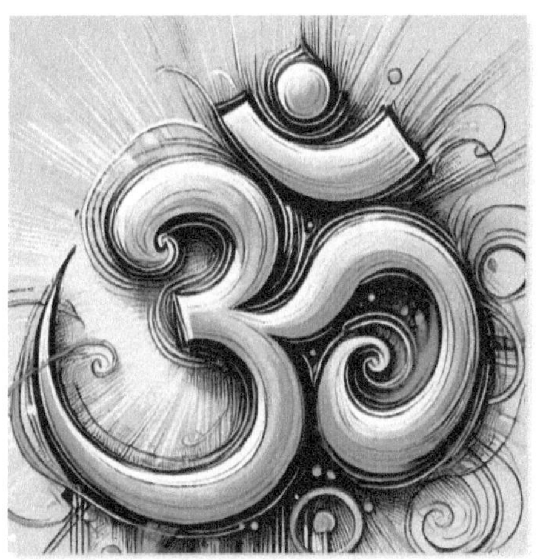

4

Mind-field

Now we realize that the mind plays a dominant role in health and disease. While we recognize stress as the main driver of physical and mental dis-eases, the engine underneath stress is a stockpile of emotions that is constantly fueling stress. We all seem to be struggling in this mindfield as we go about our daily activities. Even though we are quite familiar, it is worthwhile to put a lens on them and note how they connect with stress and impact our goal of happiness at both individual and social level.

Fear

Fear is a strong feeling that shrinks, paralyzes and shuts us down. It rises when a threat to life is perceived. It can be normal and life saving in some situations. For example, finding oneself suddenly in the midst of a fire or face to face with a predatory animal. However, it must pass to enable positive action and restore security. Fear becomes problematic when it starts predominating and staying in perpetuity.

When we live in a constant state of fear its freezing action halts the flow of vital energy. Anxiety prevails and simultaneously our strength and resistance, also referred to as immunity, reduces. We become easy prey for destructive forces including pathogenic germs. This can play havoc with the physiology of the body - putting the nervous system on overdrive, increasing stress that can cause diseases and in some cases, death.

In order to stay healthy it is therefore important to recognize fear that is abnormal and eliminate it. Worry, mistrust, suspicion, and doubt are all variations of fear. They play as much on the individual as on societal level. When we structure things at home and in society with rules and policies that breed emotional variants of fear we increase stress at different levels. The outcome is disease, depression and misery.

Happiness lives where there is trust and a sense of freedom. Trust is in fact liberating. It grants us

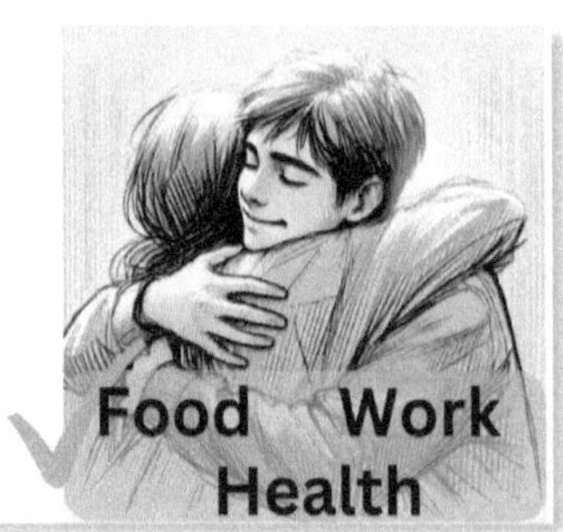

freedom. Our main fear is insufficiency in food, health and work. It stands to reason the primary antidote to fear is trust we have these. Imagining the worse - scarcity of all kinds- is a trick of the mind and it seems to plague policy-makers. We have to realize nature provides for all as long as we take care its resources. We can take charge of our health in many ways. That is what this book is about.

Once we see through the fear trick, take charge of our thoughts, adopt techniques in policy that support a clean environment, fear is easily defused. The secret is to allow only positive feelings to flow. Happiness flows in automatically.

Anger

Anger is one letter short of 'danger.' Just as an alcoholic looses self-control and is capable of endangering both the self and others, so is a person in anger. It is common to see its display - on the road right upto the parliament. There is depletion of good sense and the mind turns completely wayward. The aftermath of anger is not restoration of harmony but enhanced misery depending on what violence the enraged person unleashes. Anger expresses itself in various degrees of intensity from impatience to all out fury. No level is beneficial and the output universally is only destruction.

The antidote to anger is self-control by immediately turning attention to anger itself rather than dwelling on what appears to be the cause of it. Many times anger is rooted in fear. If that fear is defused as discussed above, anger also disappears. When you feel anger rising, a useful strategy is to distract the mind elsewhere and replace it with the other thoughts and qualities we can engender. We will discuss these in the following chapters.

Self Pity

Self pity is a festering condition wherein the person imagines him/herself as a victim that has been dealt unfair hands. The person who self-pities looks around at everyone with disdain. All cheer and self-drive towards improvement is therefore blocked. This results in a murky outlook and continual low spirits which means the cells in the body vibrate at very low frequency that dampen and push us into dis-ease.

Self pity can strike both the poor and wealthy alike. The only way out is to snap out of it and bring a determined shift in one's thought patterns. It is said self pity can be as damaging to the heart as smoking 20 cigarettes daily. If we wish to get on the road to joy, the way to self-pity must be blocked by being kind to oneself, believing we are loved and that our needs are met. We will be surprised by how our mind falsely leads us to 'think' otherwise. All we have to do is change the thoughts.

Envy

Envy is a combination of anger and self-pity. Anger because there is resentment somebody else possesses the thing we desire, and self pity because we feel inadequate and denied of it.

Envy, thus has negative effects on both mental and physical health. A few notches of intensity added, it turns into a more powerful negative force - jealousy. Both stem from comparison with others and looking at what they have which we don't.

This approach lowers self-esteem and creates anxiety that in turn can manifest in sleep disruption, cardio-vascular issues, digestive disturbances and mental problems like depression and mood disorders. Conditions that are distant from the state we really aspire for happiness.

The solution is clear as daylight and fairly easy to implement if we want to. Rather than focus on what we lack, we simply need to express gratitude for what we have. It is OK to harbor ambitions but setting goals and steering positively towards them is a better strategy- one that is in alignment with happiness.

If we think clearly we will undoubtedly accept that fear, anger, self pity, envy, and other negative emotions make us vulnerable to illness. They all are expressed one way or another by heart rate increase, increased or shortness of breath, irregular blood flow, sweating, chills, trembling muscles, digestive changes and disordered physiological functions.

Though we might justify their use in some moments, mentioning as an excuse our weakness and less evolved state, it is undeniable that they only result in waste and loss. The impact is felt on both body and spirit.

We are better off in short *and* long-term by adopting a positive attitude and moving determinedly towards our goal, believing in our aptitude.

An often neglected aspect in 'scientific' thinking is divine grace. Our spirit though not proven or identified in any shape or form by current scientific instruments, is undeniably real. It intuitively, if not logically, forms a part of this divinity and derives strength from it. It is time we stepped up and accepted this without flinching or feeling diffident.

Time-tested, venerable scriptures of India (and in other cultures) are filled with odes to divine energy. This energy establishes irrefutably the path to happiness. It is also the place wherefrom the entire natural world we see around us emanates. It is time to accept many intuitively understood universal principles for our own benefit so we can possibly attain what we fervently seek - happiness.

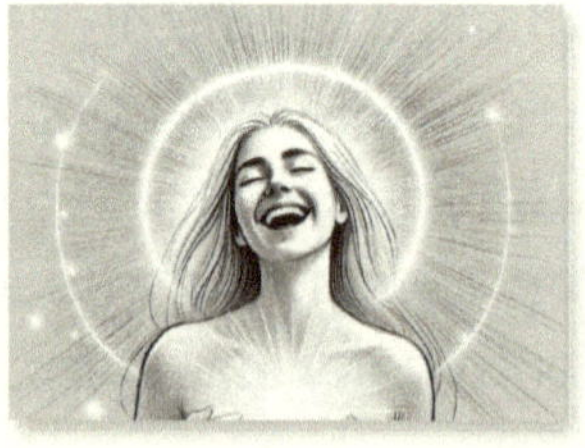

5

Pillars of Bliss

Patanjali Yoga Sutras
We do not have to research and reinvent the formula that ensures happiness. *Maharishi Patanjali* outlined it for us centuries ago and called it *Chittaprasadanam* i.e blissful mind technique.

Even today, in the age of quick fixes *this* is the antidote to everything which pulls us away from our true blissful nature. If the two - our inherent state of bliss and how we actually behave in the world on a daily basis - do not align, disharmony is created in our mind and body. If the disturbance persists for long, the mind ultimately loses its potential and instead of working *for*, it starts working *against* us. In that case, the road back to peace is not lost but becomes more arduous.

Fast-paced lifestyle and the resulting stress cause us to behave in ways that keeps creating imbalance but in *Chittaprasadanam*, Maharshi Patanjali gives us clues to align ourselves with what is our true nature. He lists four primary and universal virtues that we need to foster.

1. *Maitri* {Friendship
2. *Karuna* {Compassion
3. *Mudita* {Joy
4. *Upekshanam* {Indifference

When faced with choices that are opposite, it is up to us to choose the one that takes us closer to our fundamental disposition of bliss.

There are several distractions in daily life, but the whole point is not to let them prevail or persist. The four primary virtues of *Maharishi Patanjali* hold the key to brushing them aside and as a result reduce anxiety, stress and depression. They may appear as cliché but they work if implemented. Why not give them a try if they help us restore balance within and gain better understanding and acceptance of people and situations?

Maitri {Friendship

A friendly attitude helps us in accepting a person for 'what is' rather than demanding 'what should be.' It helps us cultivate a position of unconditional acceptance of the uniqueness in everyone and celebrate imperfections. Friendship gives a chance to further the understanding necessary for learning and personal growth because it instils trust, openness and better communication that works both ways. When we present our point of view to others, including family members, as a friend we can expect greater receptivity. After a certain age it is perhaps a better idea to treat one's children as friends too. This approach allows us to accept our own shortcomings and better, helps us surmount them. Engaging positively increases confidence and self-esteem in everyone involved. Being friendly means being empathetic which draws people and encourages strong family and community ties. Harmony and happiness are thus bound to flow.

Karuna{Compassion

Compassion is an important tool for spiritual and personal growth. When we show compassion to all life we become sympathetic observers and

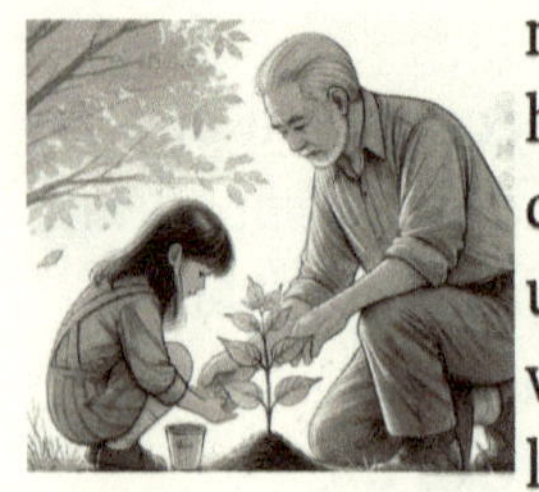

naturally less judgmental. This helps in building bridges, developing emotional understanding and connection with all involved at deeper levels than even friendship. We become more gentle with people and careful in the way we use and interact with natural resources.

It mends hearts of those wounded or less fortunate and opens those that tend to hide behind rigid and silent walls (often times our own children). More than often compassion is instrumental in bringing transformation subtly yet profoundly. We certainly become accepting of people but as importantly, of ourselves and difficult situations we face. It makes us less prone to anger and aggression. *Karuna* is a universal language with dynamic and active force.

Mudita} Joy

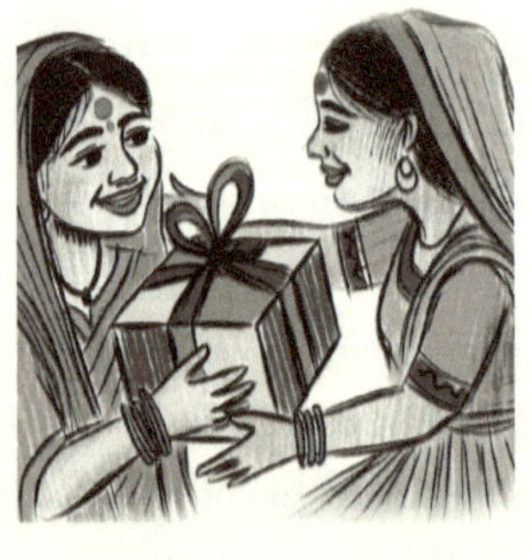

Mudita is pure, unadulterated stream of joy that flows - happiness by itself, completely devoid of self-interest. It is easy to feel joy at ones successes and accomplishments but feeling the same way for others is what brings a notable shift towards our inherent nature. Being genuinely happy for others leads to vital changes in our own mental peace and wellbeing. It is a state of high energy akin to the emotion a parent feels towards their child's triumphs. Parents selflessly give with no expectations which builds resilience and strength to face difficult circumstances. Likewise, radiating joy for everyone opens pathways that help in navigating life creatively with a sense of ease, draws positivity towards ourselves, bringing us closer to the blissful state of being.

Upeksha} Indifference

It might appear counter-intuitive but staying undisturbed or unperturbed (*Upeksha*) in day-to-day situations that might be happy, painful, successful or unfortunate maintains harmony in our *Chitta* or mind. Not reacting with anger, wailing aloud in grief, or jumping in joy but staying indifferent when faced with corresponding situations is an expression of a balanced state of mind.

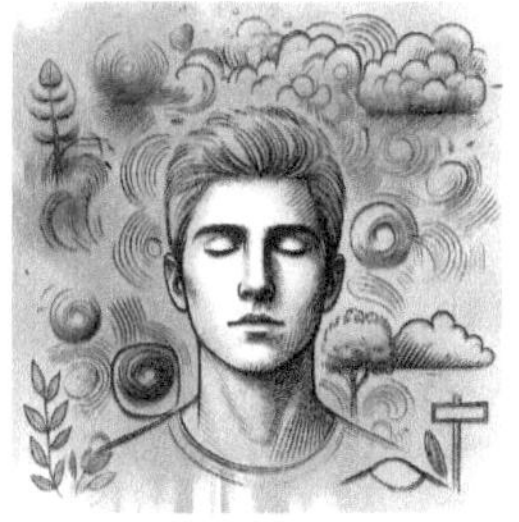

Notwithstanding the seeming difficulty in maintaining emotional stability always, this approach is most helpful in trying situations. It turns opposition around and leads to more favorable pathways. Reacting aggressively on the other hand, oftentimes escalates situations, oftentimes to irretrievable tragedy.

In a mechanical, tumultuous pace of life, developing *upeksha* towards people who are critical and judgmental is a pre-requisite on the path of peaceful living and spiritual happiness.

Inculcating the virtues prescribed by Sage Patanjali holds the secret to lasting happiness, contentment, and peace. When we function from a place of friendship, compassion, joy and indifference, every interaction and experience becomes meaningful and up-lifting. It fills life with connections, pleasure, and profound purpose. We are then able to maximize the potential of both our body and mind.

The Bhagavadgita

In the *Bhagavadgita* the entire sixteenth chapter is devoted to how we can make the mind work to its maximum potential. It distinguishes between qualities that are divine and those that are not. The benchmark for separating the two qualities is not any ethical standard but the final goal of life which is reaching a state of oneness or bliss.

Societal norms, cultural yardsticks and judicial canons are inadequate in describing the virtuousness or divinity of any action. Actions become acceptable or not solely on account of their relevance to the ultimate goal of life. If there is total harmony and relevance with the final attainment, that attitude, conduct, behaviour, thought and feeling is right, divine, and moral. If it opposes and pushes us away from the goal, it becomes unethical, immoral, not divine. That thought, word or action must, in that case, be shunned and discarded.

There are virtuous qualities that if nurtured, align us with the ultimate goal and help in sifting out inappropriate thoughts, conduct and deeds as described in the Gita.

It stands to reason there are qualities that have the opposite effect - pushing us farther from the goal. It is a matter of duty to try and imbibe the goal-aligning values even though they might seem like impractical ideals and inapplicable at the moment, while conducting our daily affairs in the world. It is befitting to remember that our goal is not short term pleasure but lasting, long-term happiness. That goal is attained from embracing these qualities and are equally valuable in

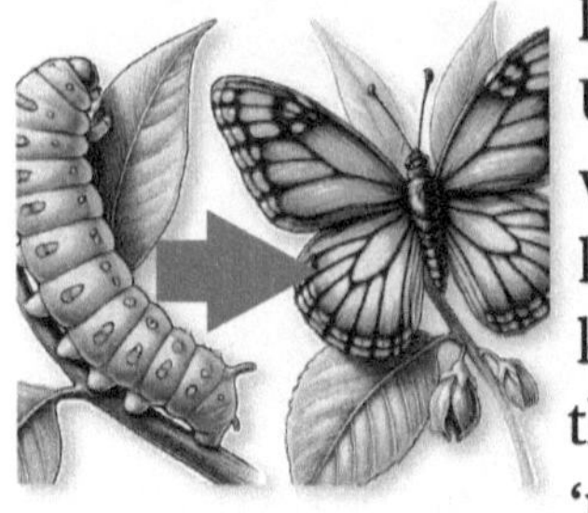

keeping misery away. Undoubtedly, the journey will be long and slow but keeping the goal in sight is key. Here is a quick run-through of the divine and 'un-divine' qualities.

DIVINE QUALITIES

The divine qualities are not simply aspirational. They must become our character. They are meritorious and define us as humans. Some appear synonymous or flowing from each each other. Some of them are therefore listed separately and others have been fused.

Abhayaṁ, or living in fearlessness is born of inner contentment. When we constantly live in a state of wanting and build relationships based on interest, we live in a state of anxiety or fear. Our desires and the thought of losing what we have underpin fear. Even as we spend time in meeting our necessities, we need to simultaneously inculcate desirelessness. The way to achieve that, however ludicrous or difficult it might seem, is by detaching emotions from material goals or outcomes. Ambition is often mistaken with

194

desire. We can be ambitious about material comfort but it *can* be delinked from desire. In that state we will find ourselves become daring and fearless.

Everything that has the attribute of truth imparts clarity of perception, radiance, and inward satiety. Hence, we have to **follow *sattva guna*,** or that which manifests the or qualities of truth and establishes us the wisdom of God. What is truth? That is learnt by exercising discrimination or sense of discernment and pursuing true knowledge.

Concomitantly we have to exercise '***Damah***,' or learn to restrain the organs of knowledge and action. The organs of knowledge are the five sense organs through which we perceive and learn about the world around - eyes, ears, nose, tongue and skin. The five organs of action are ones though which we interact and respond to the world and include our hands, feet, mouth, reproductive and elimination organs. Thus the goal should be restrain from indulgence, seeking unproductive knowledge, and displaying negative repossess. Let us instead direct energies productively elsewhere.

Dānaṁ is developing a charitable nature. Sharing a

part of what we have extends the idea of self and family. It brings into our realm of responsibility caring for those around us. This nurtures a feeling of connection and oneness with all creation.

Svādhyāyaḥ is self-directed study that keeps the mind orderly and reins in the distracting influence of sensory organs which take it adrift and away from the goal of maintaining harmony and attaining bliss. Study of the natural world and more importantly sacred scriptures and keeping company of saints and saintly people forms part of *svadhyayah*.

Ārjavam is straightforwardness - speak what we think and act what we say. It is contrary to a crooked conduct wherein we think one thing, say a second and, practice a third thing.

Other divine qualities listed for emulation include ***Ahimsa*** or practicing non-violence towards all living beings; ***Akrodhaḥ*** or freedom from anger and not losing control at any time; ***Tyāgaḥ*** which 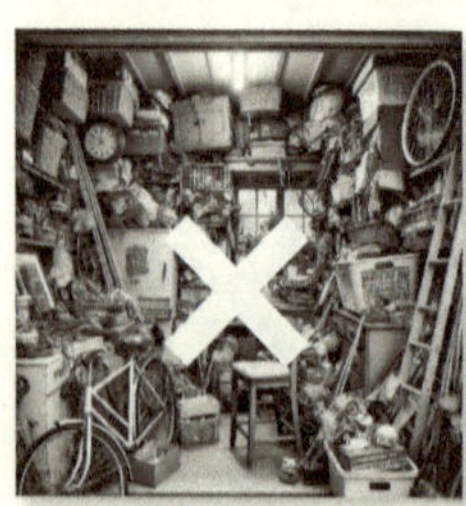 is choosing to live a simple, frugal life. We abstain from accumulating property and wealth beyond what is essential for our minimal comfortable existence; ***Śāntiḥ*** is being inwardly calm, composed and serene; *Hrīḥ* is feeling shame in the presence of things that are forbidden. It is automatic repulsion from actions and thoughts that are contrary to elevated living.

Mārdavaṁ is softness in speech, behaviour, conduct, and movement. Everything is done gently without getting irritated with anyone.

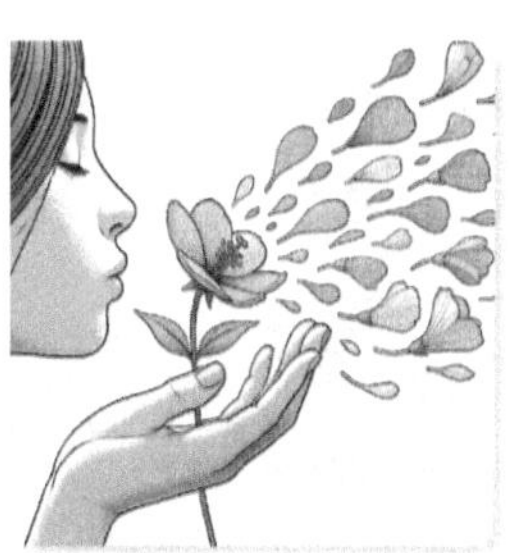

Tejaḥ is vigour, energy, and strength in the body with immense capacity for action. An indefatigable frame of body and mind rise effortlessly as a consequence of proper food habits, lifestyle and imbibing these divine qualities.

Kṣama is forgiveness. We do not try to wreak vengeance on someone who commits a mistake. Likewise we desist from dwelling over weaknesses and instead focus on strengths and good points of everyone. We be kindhearted.

Dhrtiḥ is determination to achieve our goal without slackening our effort. Staying steadfast irrespective of circumstances is an expression of determination as also affirming presence of divine qualities in oneself. Good outcomes, a happy mind and spirit flow in the face of such determination.

Śaucam is purity, both internal and external. Keeping the body clean with right choices and our environment pure and unsullied is essential for physical and spiritual prosperity.

Nātimānitā is living with no expectation of receiving regard, respect and adulation from people. Instead of wanting we should give respect to others. If we appreciate everyone, it will automatically flow back to us.

'UNDIVINE' QUALITIES
After the list of values to clothe ourselves in, here is a list we must disconnect from. Evidently they are opposite of the above mentioned noble characteristics.

Abhimāna is being intensely arrogant, egotistic and self-conscious. It is revealed in both thought and behavior. For example believing everyone is thinking of us when nobody is doing so. Constantly looking in the mirror and demonstrating excessive fondness for oneself.

Both divine and 'undivine' qualities are characterizations of human beings and apply equally to all. It is interesting how easy it is to see the *rakshasa* or demonic qualities, more and more as we get entrenched in modernism. We notice them in newspapers, social media platforms, and in media stories that love to focus and report on them. We also observe them in marketplaces, bus stands, railway stations, and other public places.

It is remarkable that the Bhagavadgita provided a comprehensive description of qualities we must nurture to ensure harmony and growth thousands of years ago. Recognizing the universality and timelessness of these qualities the Gita also provided for our benefit, an efficacious route to securing peace and happiness, if we so desire. The choice of the path is ours to make.

Purely in terms of physical health, since most diseases are psychosomatic, which means they originate in mind impulses, emulation of good qualities which are higher frequency vibrations translate into healthy cells, keeping us in fine fettle. Contrary to this, bad qualities which constitute low frequency vibrations, lead to ill-health. All the qualities discussed involve the mind which has the ability to operate at a higher level in choosing the virtuous qualities or drop to a lower level and befriend the demons. Either choice will determine what frequency our body cells vibrate in and consequently if we stay disease free.

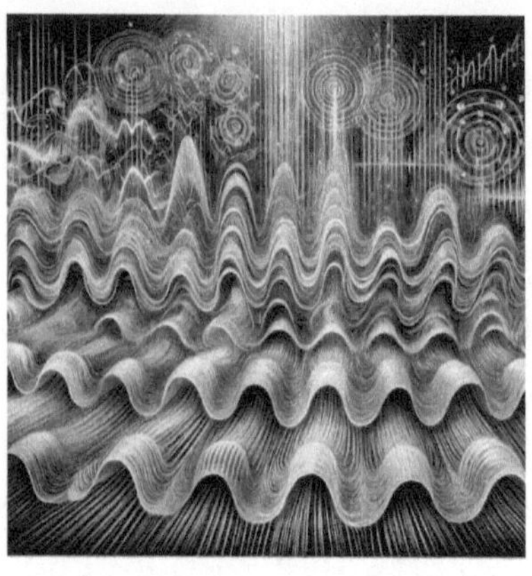

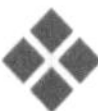

6

Placebo, Nocebo

Typically used in medical research and controlled studies, placebo is a substance (for example sugar pills), given to patients that has no real therapeutic value but the belief or perception that they are receiving medication leads to a real improvement or symptom relief. The person is then said to have experienced a placebo effect. Similarly nocebo effect occurs when negative perception or expectations of a treatment actually leads to adverse experiences and worsening of symptoms even though the treatment itself is harmless.

Both placebo and nocebo effects involve conditioning by the mind and highlights its powerful role in health and healing. The 'placebo' effect demonstrates how positive thinking can improve treatment outcomes. The 'nocebo' effect suggests that negative thinking will have a damaging effect. These effects manifest all the time in our lives. Let us take examples to see how they play out in real life.

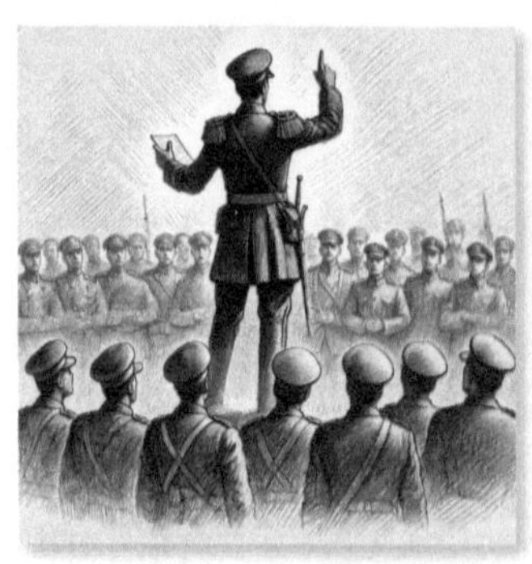 A general in the army encourages his soldiers saying - 'the enemy is less powerful, we can finish them, let us go forward, victory will be ours, the enemy cannot face us.' The army wins. Imagine the outcome if he offered suggestions in a negative way- 'the enemy is very strong, we have no chance, we may get defeated.' The result will be defeat.

Cells as Our Country

In a country it is the responsibility of the country head to take care of the needs of the people if there is to be peace, order and happiness. If we consider our body as a country then all the cells in the body are its people. As a country head we have to take care of all the cells, all the time. But are we doing our job?

When someone smiles, we can see that the smile lights the entire face. It is not just in the lips. In the same way, if someone is angry it is expressed in the entire body. This happens because every cell of the body reacts to the emotion.

Cells are basic building blocks of the body. Trillions of cells together make a body. Surprisingly every cell is an independent unit. However, all of them cooperate, coordinate, and work together as a symphony.

There is a rule book in every cell - all the instructions necessary for building and maintaining an organism. This genetic information is called human genome. Mentioned in the Vedas and yogic scriptures centuries ago, it is now understood by modern science that the genetic code in the cells can be reprogrammed. Placebo and nocebo effects is one proof of this.

We know that the child in a womb responds to the mother and gets programmed by her actions and moods. The ancient custom of *Garbh Sanskar* or preparation of motherhood, is based on practices during pregnancy that ensures physical, emotional and spiritual

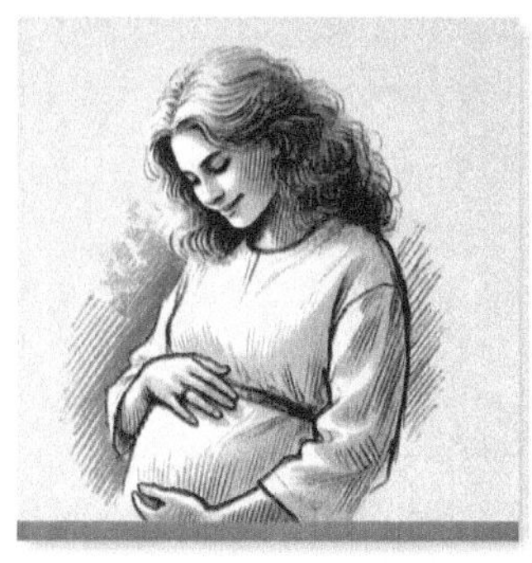

203

well being of both the mother and the developing fetus.

If *Garbh Sanskar* was not followed during pregnancy the child still has the opportunity to reprogram his or her cells for more desirable outcomes. Scientists are now experimenting with 'gene editing' and professing that our body cells listen to us and wait for orders. We have to manage them as a captain through our thoughts. What are we doing?

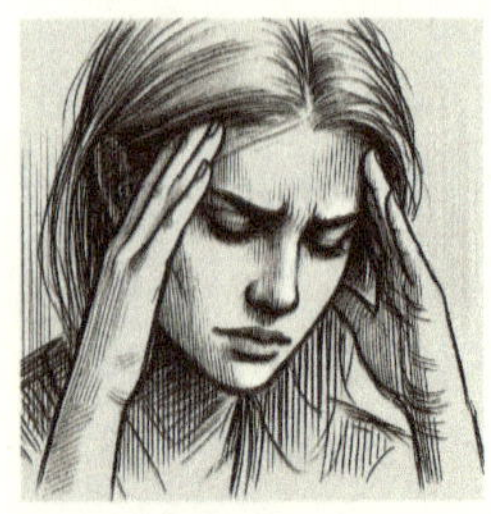

We think and feel negatively most of the time and this message hits the cells, making them dysfunctional. We start our day with complaints about everything - financial matters, children, job, business, and health. We feel overwhelmed and exasperated. Consequently these thoughts affect the body.

Some imagine they have a serious illness and with self talk give autosuggestion to their cells. The cells receive this suggestion, believe it and respond accordingly. In case of headache if we repeatedly

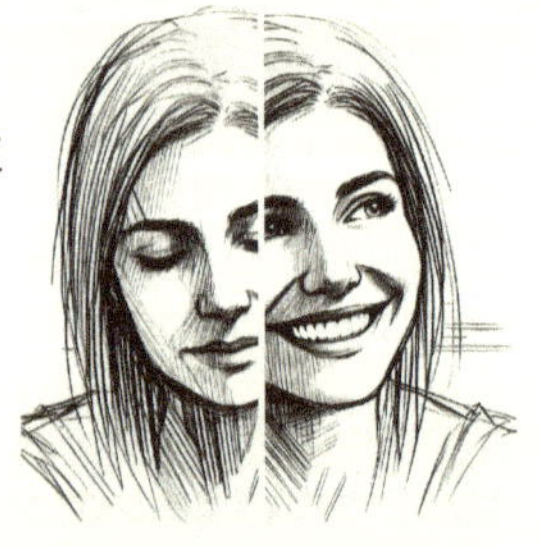

say that the head is hurting intensely and no tablet is working, the headache will likely become unbearable.

When it comes to addiction, addicts believe they cannot live without the substance - be it tea, coffee, sweets, alcohol or drugs. That is why de-addiction treatment works only when the addict is convinced (s)he wants to get rid of the addiction. Doctors know without the person's desire to get well, the medicine will not work and healing will fail.

On the other hand, a positive thought can change things for the better. If you believe you can digest anything you eat (clearly from the good choices category), then the cells in the stomach respond accordingly and help in the digestion.

When we meet people we normally ask each other how we feel. A positive response itself helps because the body cells listen to the autosuggestion.

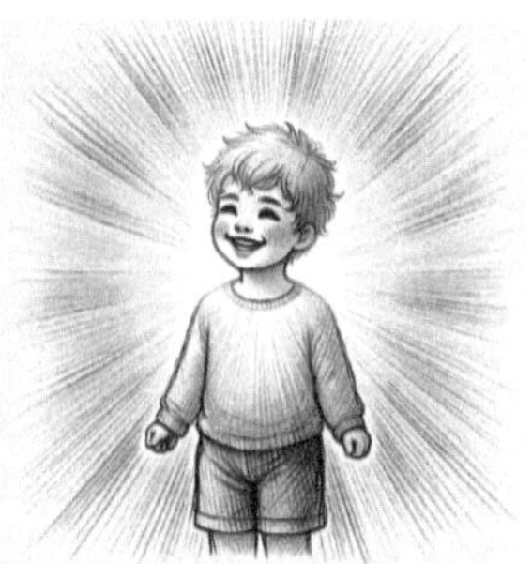

A surge of happy feeling experienced when one wins a lottery, gets a big hike in salary or recovers a written off loan, spreads to all our body cells. They get energized with the buoyant vibrations and work efficiently with enthusiasm, removing all toxins, maintaining good health in the body. Even though these instances are not part of daily occurrence we can make a habit to react positively to every situation and transmit healthful vibrations to our cells. This indeed is the method, a powerful one at that, to staying healthy.

When a child fails in an exam, instead of responding with negative comments that discredit and debase, we can elect to encourage, motivate and build confidence so future efforts can lead to success. The result will surely be positive.

Being positive does not mean we lie about facts and fool ourselves. Looking at the above examples, the general's army may be the smaller one compared to the enemy's, the digestive system may be problematic or the child doesn't in fact have the potential to score a success. The following story of a deaf frog will illustrate the relevance and strength in positive thinking and equally so in warding off the negative.

A group of frogs were trying to leap out of a well. Some tried but failed. So they related their unsuccessful efforts to other frogs and discouraged them saying it was a wasted effort. The well was too deep to hop out 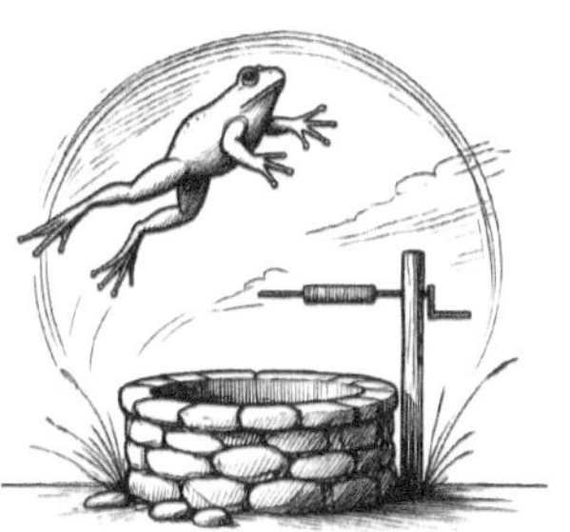 of. The other frogs listened. Some who were trying stopped and others who hadn't even made a single effort, went away without making any attempt. But in the group there was a deaf frog which did not listen to the negative suggestions. It kept trying and finally succeeded in making that one leap to liberation.

So what are we to do? Our timeless yogic texts and today even scientists, say: Give good suggestions or constant affirmations to cells. In case of ill-health in any part of the body, send positive message to the cells to repair and cure the disease. The cells will respond positively. Good thoughts are as essential as good food.

There is no cost involved in reprogramming ourselves and giving affirmations. Remember, "sooner or later, the man who wins is the man who *thinks* he can." This is how the placebo effect works. Never indulge the nocebo effect and try daily to make the placebo technique work for you.

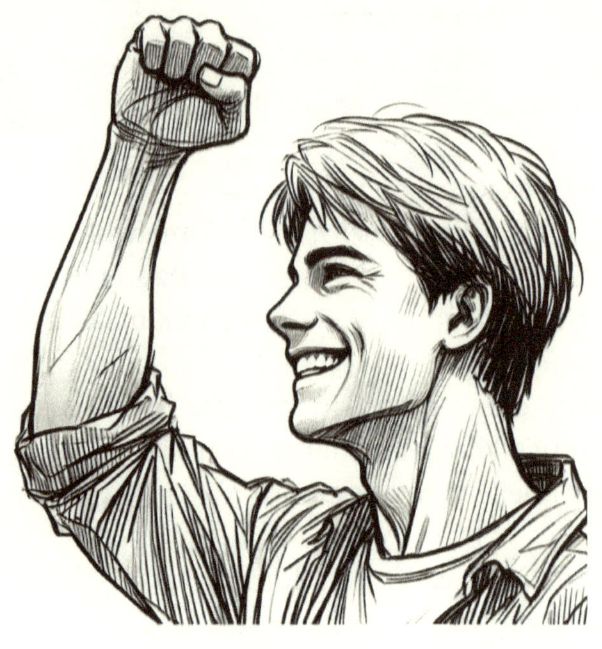

7

Happiness Forever

We all try to be happy and resort to objects, events, and changing circumstances. To give examples we buy material things, take vacations, plan celebrations, take a new job, or move to a new place. Noticeably, all methods are external and short lived. We have seen in chapter 5 that our real nature is '*Ananda*' or joy. We can be in a state of lasting happiness even as we follow the necessary dictates of the world. We read in chapter five about developing right qualities and attitude. In this final chapter is the technique of being in the state of '*Ananda*' all the time. Really so.

In the *Bhagavadgita* the word '*samatva*' is mentioned repeatedly. The simple meaning of '*samatva*' is even-mindedness or equanimity, i.e. accepting both the good and bad in the same manner. *That* is the state of real happiness or

Ananda. Is it possible to receive our fortune and misfortune similarly? Yes, it is.

Daily Life Situations
In daily life there are many situations that we regard as good or bad depending upon our perception.

As mentioned earlier, if a child fails the exam we feel hopeless about their future. However, we forget rigid schooling may not be suited for every child and there are multiple pathways to growth, learning, and success. There are many instances in history where after dropping out or even being expelled from school, the person achieved global fame and success.

Albert Einstein, Thomas Edison were both considered slow and 'unable to learn' by their schools. Kalidasa was uneducated and ridiculed. He went on to become one of the greatest Sanskrit poet and playwright. There are plentiful examples in the West of people not schooled as per the 'system' who nevertheless went on become trailblazers. Ancient India sages followed a different route to wisdom and shared their learnings which even modern science is yet to catch up to. They include Panini, Patanjali,

Valmiki, Aryabhatta, Chanakya, Charaka, and Sushruta.

There is a well known story of a famous sweets brand owner in Andhra Pradesh. He failed in matriculation (10th class) exam which was a big shock for his parents. They dreamt of a good job in the railways for their son. But his uncle thought differently. With the uncle's help the young man joined a sweet shop as an assistant. The rest of the story is that the boy went on to establish his own brand name and prospered to become a business magnate in the sweets industry. Was his school failure bad?

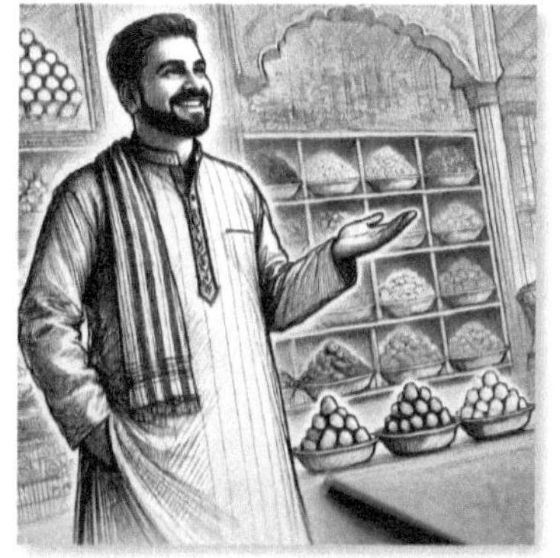

Many parents work their backs off in bringing up children who often times leave and sometimes treat the parents indifferently or poorly. Those times the parents wish they did not have children. But in either situation - is having or not having children - really bad ?

A bank manager in one area dismissed an attendant for his misdemeanor. The attendant took it as a life challenge and started a *pan* shop in front of the bank. In due course he flourished as a businessman. Not treating his job dismissal as a failure but merely as a change in direction he did the best he could with a positive attitude and tasted success.

When people praise us, we feel elated. When we are criticized we feel dejection. If we examine closely, it is actually *our* response that makes us happy or unhappy. Though criticism is an opportunity to correct ourselves, the response we give is totally in our control. We can remain unaffected as long as we have '*samatva*'.

Routinely we say we are not lucky. We feel our stars are not in correct alignment. Whether that is true or not, we still have it in our hands to respond to our situations. Our best choice in dealing with hard times is to remain in '*samatva*' state and continue being positive.

There is no good or bad. Ignorance and rigidity in the way of seeing things is the cause of unhappiness. Our thoughts, opinions and ideas on life which are grooved in our mind keep us ignorant. Now with the knowledge outlined in these chapters we have a chance to step out of our grooves and reprogram our mind. We can change ourself at any time. It is never late. Knowing our nature is *Sat Chit Ananda* we can get closer to it and be happy, forever.

❖

Bibliography

- Publications of Bihar School of Yoga, India.
- Siri Jagattu publication, Padmasri Dr.Khadar Vali, Millet Man of India.
- Health in your Hands, Devendra Vora on Acupressure and other Natural TherapiesHealth in your Hands, Devendra Vora on Acupressure and other Natural Therapies.
- Naturopathy Medicine, https://www.naturesmedicinethroughtime.org/
- American Journal of Clinical Nutrition; https://ajcn.nutrition.org
- jstor.org
- Integrative Medicine; https://www.acam.org/page/TheVoiceARCHIVE
- Traditional Medicine; https://www.who.int/initiatives/who-global-traditional-medicine-centre
- https://www.who.int/news-room/questions-and-answers/item/traditional-medicine
- https://www.sciencedirect.com/science/article/abs/pii/S0899900708004085
- Herbs in Oral Health Care; https://pubmed.ncbi.nlm.nih.gov/38290997/
- Diet for a Small Planet, Frances Moore Lappe
- https://www.naturalnews.com/2024-10-18-sandalwood-natures-fragrant-shield-against-cancer.html
- Giloy: https://www.nature.com/articles/s41598-024-53176-z
- https://www.sciencedirect.com/science/article/abs/pii/S1369527424000705
- Yoga & Naturopathy for Hypothyroid; https://www.sciencedirect.com/science/article/abs/pii/S2212958824001216

- https://www.cdc.gov
- http://www.health.harvard.edu/
- http://www.bbc.com/news/health
- Microwaves & Pathogenic Bacteria; https://www.sciencenews.org/article/some-bacteria-flourish-microwave-ovens
- Tulsi Benefits: https://onlinelibrary.wiley.com/doi/10.1155/2024/8895039
- Fulfilling the Promise of Microbiomics to Revolutionize Medicine; https://pmc.ncbi.nlm.nih.gov/articles/PMC4809425/
- Loving Yourself to Great Health, *Louise Hay, Ahlea Khadro, Heather Dane*
- Herbal Antivirals, *Stephen Harrod Buhner*
- *Planta Medica*
- Phytomedicine Journal; Wound healing with Flavonoids & Curcumin: *https://www.sciencedirect.com/science/article/abs/pii/S0944711321001793; https://www.sciencedirect.com/science/article/abs/pii/S0141813019356168*
- Phytotherapy Research; *Polyphenols: A concise overview on the chemistry, occurrence, and human health, July 2019*
- Journal of Medicinal Plants Research; *https://academicjournals.org/journal/JMPR*
- Advances in Therapy Journal;*Medicinal Plants in the Indian Traditional Medicine and Current Practices; Aug 31, 2023*
- Journal of Medicinal Food; *Ginger–An Herbal Medicinal Product with Broad Anti-Inflammatory Actions; 20 July 2005*
- Journal of Medicinal Plants Research
- Alternative Medicine Review; https://altmedrev.com/
- Natural Product Communication
- Healing through Gerson Way, Charlotte Gerson, Beata Bishop

- Evidence based Complementary and Alternative
  Medicine Journal
- fao.org/hunger; State of Food Security & Nutrition

Note

Information contained in this book is provided for general and educational purposes only. Even though they might not be well known they are based on timeless traditions, practiced by cultures across the globe, many of which are well documented in studies done by leading research institutes of the world. The authors encourage the reader to make their own health care decisions, guided by their own research and in partnership with a specialist or qualified healthcare professional. The authors assume no responsibility or liability for any adverse effects or consequences resulting from use of the book. Readers are encouraged to exercise their own judgment and discretion in applying the content to their personal circumstances.